Endovascular Intervention: Today and Tomorrow

Series Editor

Frank J. Criado, MD

Volume 2

Endovascular Intervention: Today and Tomorrow

Series Editor
Frank J. Criado, MD
Director, Center for Vascular Intervention
Chief, Division of Vascular Surgery
Union Memorial Hospital/MedStar Health
Baltimore, MD

Volume 2

Endovascular Therapy for Atherosclerotic Renal Artery Stenosis:

Present and Future

Edited by

Michael R. Jaff, DO, FACP, FACC
Director, Vascular Medicine
Co-Director, Vascular Diagnostic Laboratory
The Heart and Vascular Institute
Morristown, New Jersey

Futura Publishing Company
Armonk, NY

Library of Congress Cataloging-in-Publication Data

Endovascular therapy for atherosclerotic renal artery stenosis : present and future / edited by Michael R. Jaff.
    p. ; cm. — (Endovascular intervention ; v.2)
    Includes bibliographical references and index.
    ISBN 0-87993-470-0 (alk. paper)
    1. Renal artery obstruction. 2. Stents (Surgery). 3. Kidney—Blood-vessels. 4. Endoscopy. I. Jaff, Michael R. II. Series.
    [DNLM: 1. Renal Artery Obstruction—surgery. 2. Endoscopy. 3. Renal Artery—pathology. 4. Stents. 5. Vascular Surgical Procedures. WJ 368 E56 2001]
    RD575 .E534 2001
    617.4'61—dc21

                                    2001040233

Published by
Futura Publishing Company
135 Bedford Road
Armonk, New York 10504

LC#: 2001040233
ISBN#: 0-87993-470-0

Every effort has been made to ensure that the information in this book is as up to date and accurate as possible at the time of publication. However, due to the constant developments in medicine, neither the author, nor the editors, nor the publisher can accept any legal or any other responsibility for any errors or omissions that may occur.

Printed in the United States of America on acid-free paper.

Introduction

Atherosclerotic stenosis of the renal artery has become a widely discussed and debated topic in modern cardiovascular medicine. There are multiple reasons for this, including an aging population, improved imaging modalities, novel safe and effective methods of revascularization, improvement in antiplatelet therapy, and effective management of access site complications after percutaneous procedures.

Despite the intense interest in renal artery disease, there still remains great confusion about the incidence and prevalence, natural history, ideal algorithm for diagnosis, beneficial effects of revascularization, optimal methods of revascularization, and ultimately, whether or not revascularization has a positive impact on renal preservation.

This monograph is designed to explore the current thinking related to all aspects of atherosclerotic renal artery stenosis. With contributions from recognized international leaders in this field, this book represents the most comprehensive analysis of present data and experience.

Although this field is rapidly evolving, the comments made in this book explore appropriate diagnostic testing, and in-depth discussions about surgical and endovascular revascularization in atherosclerotic renal artery stenosis.

I owe a tremendous debt of gratitude to the physicians who have contributed to the success of this book. Their expertise is invaluable, and I am grateful for their input.

Michael R. Jaff, DO, FACP, FACC

Contributors

Mark C. Bates, MD, FACC   Senior Scientist Cardiovascular Research Camcare Health Education and Research Institute, Clinical Professor in Medicine, Robert C. Byrd Health Sciences Center, Charleston, WV; Clinical Professor in Medicine, Marshall University, Huntington, WV; Director, Circulatory Dynamics Laboratory, CAMC, Charleston, WV

Susan M. Begelman, MD   Department of Vascular Medicine, Cleveland Clinic Foundation, Cleveland, OH

Richard P. Cambria, MD   Associate Professor of Surgery, Division of Vascular Surgery, Massachusetts General Hospital, Boston, MA

Gerald Dorros, MD   The William Dorros-Isadore Feuer Interventional Cardiovascular Disease Foundation Ltd., Phoenix, AZ and Grafton, WI

Robert F. Fishman, MD   Cardiac Specialists of Fairfield, P.C., Director, Interventional Cardiology Fellowship Program, Bridgeport Hospital, Bridgeport, CT

Kimberley J. Hansen, MD, FACS   Professor of Surgery, Department of GeneralSurgery, Wake Forest University School of Medicine, Winston-Salem, NC

Thomas He, PhD   Biostatistician

Michael R. Jaff, DO, FACP, FACC   Director, Vascular Medicine, Co-Director, Vascular Diagnostic Laboratory, The Heart and Vascular Institute, Morristown, NJ

John L. Kaufman, MD   Division of Vascular Surgery, Massachusetts General Hospital, Boston, MA

Lynne Mathiak, RN   Assistant Medical Director, The William Dorros-Isadore Feuer Interventional Cardiovascular Disease Foundation Ltd., Phoenix, AZ and Grafton, WI

Michael McKusick, MD   Associate Professor of Medicine, Mayo Medical School, Department of Interventional Radiology, Mayo Clinic, Rochester, MN

Jeffrey W. Olin, DO   Department of Vascular Medicine, Cleveland Clinic Foundation, Cleveland, OH

Timothy C. Oskin, MD   Department of General Surgery, Wake Forest University School of Medicine, Winston-Salem, NC

Stephen R. Ramee   Ochsner Heart & Vascular Institute, New Orleans, LA

Kenneth Rosenfield, MD   Director, Vascular International Suite, Division of Vascular Medicine, St. Elizabeth Medical Center, Boston, MA

DE Strandness Jr., MD, D. Med. (Hon)   Professor of Surgery, Department of Surgery, University of Washington School of Medicine, Seattle, WA

Stephen C. Textor, MD   Professor of Medicine, Mayo Medical School, Division of Hypertension Mayo Clinic, Rochester, MN

Christopher J. White   Chairman, Department of Cardiology, Ochsner Clinic, New Orleans, LA

James M. Wong, MD   Department of General Surgery, Wake Forest University School of Medicine, Winston-Salem, NC

Contents

Atherosclerotic Renal Artery Stenosis:

Prevalence and Clinical Manifestations

Susan M. Begelman, MD and Jeffrey W. Olin, DO

Introduction

Atherosclerosis is a progressive, systemic disease and is the leading cause of death in the United States. While its effect on the coronary and carotid arteries is well recognized, involvement of the renal arteries is frequently overlooked. Atherosclerosis accounts for at least two-thirds of all renovascular lesions. However, the exact prevalence of renovascular disease is not known, despite extensive research and state-of-the-art diagnostic studies. Atherosclerotic renal artery stenosis (RAS) is a correctable cause of secondary hypertension, ischemic nephropathy, and "flash" or recurrent pulmonary edema. Therefore, early diagnosis and treatment is of vital importance to avoid premature morbidity and mortality.

Prevalence

While there are excellent prevalence data in specific patient populations (i.e., those with coronary artery disease, an aortic aneurysm, peripheral arterial disease), the prevalence of RAS in the general population is not known.

From Jaff MR (ed): *Endovascular Therapy for Atherosclerotic Renal Artery Stenosis: Present and Future*. Armonk, NY: Future Publishing Co, Inc.; ©2001.

Data on prevalence is difficult to interpret for several reasons. First, not all cases of RAS are clinically significant. Dustan et al.[1] reviewed 149 aortograms and found that approximately half of patients with $\geq$ 50% RAS did *not* have hypertension. Not all patients with RAS and hypertension have the hypertension mediated by the RAS. Some individuals have primary or essential hypertension and anatomic RAS that is independent of the hypertension. Secondly, when patients are symptomatic, the presentation is not uniform. Lastly, the prevalence of RAS changes with age, as does the prevalence of atherosclerosis elsewhere. This change, in part, reflects the progressive nature of the disease. For example, in a prospective study by Zierler et al.[2] the cumulative incidence of progression from < 60% stenosis to $\geq$ 60% stenosis was 30% at 1 year, 44% at 2 years, and 48% at 3 years. The average rate of progression from baseline was 7% per year for all categories of disease. Despite the difficulties in studying disease prevalence, estimates have been made based on examination during autopsy, reviews of unselected arteriograms of patients who undergo evaluation of atherosclerosis elsewhere (such as coronary artery disease or peripheral arterial disease), and renal artery angiography in patients in whom the physician has a high clinical suspicion for RAS.

The prevalence of atherosclerotic RAS has been reported in several autopsy series. Holley et al.[3] looked at 295 consecutive patients and found RAS (defined as $\geq$ 50% stenosis) in 53%. The prevalence increased to 74% when only those individuals older than 70 were considered. Likewise, Schwartz et al.[4] prospectively studied 154 consecutive patients at autopsy. They found RAS in 24% of all patients and in 86% of patients age 75 or older. More recently, 297 patients > 40 years old with autopsy-proven myocardial infarction were examined for evidence of atherosclerotic RAS.[5] Significant stenosis (> 75% luminal narrowing) was documented in 12% of patients. Since atherosclerosis increases with age, it makes sense that the prevalence of atherosclerotic RAS would be greater among the elderly.

Several series have looked at the prevalence of renovascular disease in patients who have atherosclerotic disease elsewhere. To determine the prevalence of RAS, we studied 395 consecutive patients who had atherosclerosis in other peripheral arteries (Table 1).[6] These patients did not have the usual clin-

Table 1.

Prevalence of Atherosclerotic RAS.
(395 Consecutive Arteriograms)

$\geq$ 50% Stenosis	AAA (n = 109)	AOD (n = 21)	LEOD (n = 189)	RAS (n = 76)
All patients	41 (38%)	7 (33%)	74 (39%)	53 (70%)*
Diabetic	6 (50%)	1 (33%)	34 (50%)**	10 (71%)
Nondiabetic	35 (36%)	6 (33%)	40 (33%)	43 (69%)*

AAA – abdominal aortic aneurysm; AOD – aortoiliac occlusive disease; LEOD – lower extremity occlusive disease; RAS – renal artery stenosis; *P < 0.001 compared to other 3 groups; **P < 0.022 compared to nondiabetic patients with LEOD. From reference #6.

ical clues to suggest RAS. The data demonstrates that the frequency of atherosclerotic RAS is 38% in patients undergoing arteriography for abdominal aortic aneurysm, 33% for patients with aortoiliac occlusive disease, and 39% for patients with lower extremity occlusive disease. In addition, those patients with diabetes mellitus were as likely to have significant RAS as those without diabetes. High-grade bilateral renal artery disease was present in approximately 13% of patients. Metcalfe et al.[7] recently reported a 36.2% prevalence of RAS in a series of 218 patients who had angiograms to evaluate peripheral arterial disease. Other studies to evaluate the prevalence of RAS in patients with peripheral arterial disease have demonstrated similar rates (Table 2).[8]

Harding et al.[9] performed abdominal aortography at the time of cardiac catheterization in 1,235 patients and found that 30% had renal artery disease. Only half of the patients had documented luminal narrowing of at least 50%. Ramirez et al.[10] demonstrated a 13.7% prevalence of RAS at the time of coronary catheterization in 102 consecutive patients.

Some studies report disease prevalence for individuals in whom there are clinical clues to suggest the presence of RAS. This increases the pretest probability for underlying RAS and, as one would suspect, increases the prevalence of the disease. For example, in the study done at our institution described above, 70% of patients with a suggestive history of RAS were found to have significant disease.[6] Traditionally, this has not been true when considering individual characteristics such as hypertension. It is thought that 20% of adults have hypertension (defined as a blood pressure $\geq$ 140/90 mmHg). This number increases to 50% when considering individuals older than 60.[11] Although renovascular hypertension is a common secondary cause of hypertension, it is estimated to be the etiologic factor in only 0.2% to 5% of patients with hypertension.[12,13] The prevalence of renovascular hypertension was found to be high in patients with accelerated or malignant hypertension.[14]

Several series have looked at the prevalence of bilateral RAS (Table 3).[6,15] In the 319 patients reported in 6 different studies, 44% of patients had bilateral RAS. In patients with an atrophic kidney, there is a prevalence of RAS in the contralateral normal sized kidney in approximately 59%.[16,17]

Table 2.

Prevalence of Atherosclerotic RAS in Patients with Peripheral Arterial Disease.

Reference	Association	% (Total No.)
Dustan (1964)	PVD	37 (149)
Olin (1990)	PVD	39 (189)
Wilms (1990)	PVD	22 (100)
Choudhri (1990)	PVD	59 (100)
Swartbol (1992)	PVD	49 (450)
Missouris (1994)	PVD	45 (127)

From Scoble JE.[8]

Table 3.

	Prevalence of Bilateral Renal Artery Stenosis.		
	Stenotic Arteries	*Bilateral*	
Reference	*n*	*n (%)*	*Method*
Holley 1964	159	105 (66)	Autopsy
Wollenweber 1968	109	67 (61)	Arteriogram
Dean 1981	41	14 (34)	Arteriogram
Olin 1990	175	67 (38)	Arteriogram
Tollefson 1991	48	14 (29)	Arteriogram
Harding 1992	192	52 (27)	Arteriogram
Total	724	319 (44)	

Adapted from Rimmer & Gennari.[15]

Clinical Clues

The three most common presentations of atherosclerotic RAS are uncontrolled hypertension, azotemia (ischemic nephropathy), and "flash" or recurrent pulmonary edema. It is also not uncommon to discover RAS incidentally during the evaluation of some other problem. Several clinical features (Table 4)[17] have been shown to increase the likelihood of underlying RAS.

Essential hypertension usually occurs in individuals between the ages of 30 and 55. While systolic blood pressure increases with age, diastolic blood pressure usually increases up until the age of 55 and then begins to decline. Therefore, the diagnosis of RAS should be sought when patients present with hypertension younger than 30 or older than 55 years of age. RAS in the young is usually due to fibromuscular dysplasia while atherosclerosis is more often the etiology in older individuals. It is not uncommon for atherosclerotic RAS to coexist with essential hypertension. This should be considered when a patient has been well-maintained on medications and suddenly the blood pressure be-

Table 4.

**Clinical Clues to the Diagnosis of
Atherosclerotic Renovascular Disease.**

1. Onset of diastolic hypertension after the age of 55
2. Exacerbation of previously well controlled hypertension
3. Malignant hypertension
4. Resistant hypertension
5. Epigastric bruit (systolic/diastolic)
6. Unexplained azotemia
7. Azotemia while receiving ACE inhibitors
8. Atrophic kidney or discrepancy in size between the kidneys
9. Atherosclerosis elsewhere
10. Flash pulmonary edema or recurrent congestive heart failure

From Olin JW, Novick AC.[17]

comes difficult to control. Malignant or accelerated hypertension is associated with RAS. Davis et al.[14] demonstrated that the prevalence of RAS was approximately 30% in patients with grade III (accelerated hypertension) and grade IV (malignant hypertension) hypertensive retinopathy. Renal artery disease should be considered in patients who despite a multi-drug regimen with three medications each of a different pharmacologic class, do not have adequately controlled blood pressure (< 140/90 mmHg).

The physical exam is of limited help in making the diagnosis of atherosclerotic RAS. Patients with atherosclerosis elsewhere are more likely to have atherosclerotic RAS.[6,7,8] Therefore, evidence of coronary, cerebral, or peripheral arterial disease should raise one's suspicion for RAS. The presence of a systolic/diastolic bruit in the epigastrium increases the likelihood of RAS.[18] A bruit audible over the flanks occurs less often. Simon et al.[19] evaluated 175 patients with renovascular hypertension and 339 patients with essential hypertension and found that the presence of a bruit was 6 to 9 times more frequent in patients with RAS than in those with essential hypertension alone (7% essential hypertension, 41% atherosclerotic RAS, 57% fibromuscular dysplasia of the renal arteries). Other studies similarly show that the characteristic systolic/diastolic bruit is more commonly found in patients with underlying RAS due to fibromuscular dysplasia than atherosclerosis.[20,21]

Renal artery stenosis has significant deleterious effects on the kidney. Historically, the presence of an atrophic kidney was thought to be due to chronic pyelonephritis. The most common cause is now known to be due to ischemic damage from RAS. Gifford et al.[16] found that 53 of 75 (71%) hypertensive patients with a unilateral atrophic kidney had RAS. This was confirmed by pathology in 35 of 42 (83%) patients with stenotic or occluded renal arteries. A recent prospective study showed a two-year cumulative incidence of renal atrophy in a kidney with RAS to be 20.8%.[22] Likewise, RAS should also be considered in a patient with a discrepancy in kidney size.

Azotemia that cannot be explained, especially in the elderly, or azotemia related to the use of an angiotensin-converting enzyme inhibitor (ACEI) or angiotensin II antagonist increases the likelihood of underlying RAS. This is especially true in patients with bilateral disease or disease to a solitary functioning kidney. Two mechanisms have been described to explain this phenomenon. In patients with severe stenosis, there may be a critical perfusion pressure which must be maintained in order for renal function to remain normal. It has been shown that once the systemic blood pressure is lowered below this critical perfusion pressure (which is different for each patient), the glomerular filtration rate (GFR) and urine output decreases.[23] The second mechanism is specific to the use of an ACEI or angiotensin-II antagonists and can occur without significant reduction in blood pressure. Patients with bilateral RAS or stenosis of a single functioning kidney may rely on angiotensin II to maintain their GFR (especially in the volume contracted state). This occurs by constriction of the efferent arteriole which increases the transglomerular hydraulic capillary pressure. An ACEI will prevent this physiologic adaptation (efferent arteriolar constriction) and the blood will be shunted from the afferent arteriole to the efferent arteriole (thus bypassing glomerular filtration) producing acute renal failure.[17,24]

The most recent clinical association described between RAS and its presentation is that of "flash" pulmonary edema or recurrent episodes of congestive heart failure (CHF) not due to underlying ischemic cardiac disease. Pickering et al.[25] reported a series of 55 consecutive patients with symptomatic atherosclerotic RAS (hypertension and azotemia) and found a 23% prevalence of pulmonary edema. Virtually all of these patients had bilateral RAS or RAS to a solitary functioning kidney. The mechanism by which high grade bilateral RAS causes CHF has not been completely worked out. In some patients, surges in blood pressure in the presence of a noncompliant left ventricle may be the cause. Salt and water retention with associated volume expansion or direct effects of angiotensin II may also play an important role in causing CHF. It has been clearly demonstrated that renal revascularization, using either an endovascular (angioplasty or stent) or surgical approach, can decrease the severity and frequency of recurrent pulmonary edema.[26,27]

Conclusion

As the population ages and more individuals have other manifestations of atherosclerosis, the presence of atherosclerotic RAS is more commonly encountered. Awareness of the population at risk and attention to the clinical clues lead to earlier diagnosis and a greater chance that intervention will be helpful in controlling blood pressure, preventing progressive azotemia, and controlling congestive heart failure. Diagnostic modalities most frequently used include captopril stimulated renography,[28] duplex ultrasound of the renal arteries,[29] spiral computerized tomographic angiography of the renal arteries,[30] magnetic resonance angiography of the renal arteries,[31] intra-arterial digital subtraction arteriography,[32] and CO_2 angiography.[33] The choice of study is highly dependent on equipment and expertise available at one's institution. Early recognition and treatment can decrease the morbidity and mortality associated with atherosclerotic renal artery stenosis.

References

1. Dustan HP, Humphries AW, De Wolfe VG, et al. Normal arterial pressure in patients with renal arterial stenosis. *JAMA* 1964; 187:1028–1029.
2. Zierler RE, Bergelin RO, Davidson RC, et al. A prospective study of disease progression in patients with atherosclerotic renal artery stenosis. *Am J Hypertens* 1996; 9:1055–1061.
3. Holley KE, Hunt JC, Brown AL, et al. Renal artery stenosis: A clinical-pathological study in normotensive and hypertensive patients. *Am J Med* 1964; 37:14–22.
4. Schwartz CJ, White TA. Stenosis of renal artery: An unselected necropsy study. *Br Med J* 1964; 2:1415–1421.
5. Uzu T, Inoue T, Fujii T, et al. Prevalence and predictors of renal artery stenosis in patients with myocardial infarction. *Am J Kidney Dis* 1997; 29:733–738.
6. Olin JW, Melia M, Joung JR, et al. Prevalence of atherosclerotic renal artery stenosis in patients with atherosclerosis elsewhere. *Am J Med* 1990; 88:1–46N-1–51N.
7. Metcalfe W, Reid AW, Geddes CC. Prevalence of angiographic atherosclerotic renal artery disease and its relationship to the anatomical extent of peripheral vascular atherosclerosis. *Nephrol Dial Transplant* 1999; 14:105–108.

8. Scoble JE. The epidemiology and clinical manifestations of atherosclerotic renal disease. In Novick AC, Scoble J, Hamilton G (eds): **Renal Vascular Disease**. London, WB Saunders Co., Ltd., 1996, pp 303–314.
9. Harding MB, Smith LR, Himmelstein SI, et al. Renal artery stenosis: Prevalence and associated risk factors in patients undergoing routine cardiac catheterization. *J Am Soc Nephrol* 1992; 2:1608–1616.
10. Ramirez G, Bugni W, Farber SM, et al. Incidence of renal artery stenosis in a population having cardiac catheterization. *South Med J* 1987; 80:734–737.
11. Mulrow PJ. Hypertension. A worldwide epidemic. In Izzo JL Jr, Black HR (eds): **Hypertension Primer**. Baltimore, MD, Lippincott Williams & Wilkins, second edition, 1999, pp 271–273.
12. Gifford RW Jr: Evaluation of the hypertensive patient with emphasis on detecting curable causes. *Milbank Mem Fund Q* 1969, 47:170–186.
13. Svetkey LP, Helms MJ, Dunnick NR, et al. Clinical characteristics useful in screening for renovascular disease. *South Med J* 1990; 83:743–747.
14. Davis BA, Crook JE, Vestal RE, et al. Prevalence of renovascular hypertension in patients with grade III or IV hypertensive retinopathy. *N Engl J Med* 1979; 301:1273–1276.
15. Rimmer JM, Gennari FJ. Atherosclerotic renovascular disease and progressive renal failure. *Ann Intern Med* 1993; 118:712–719.
16. Gifford RW Jr, McCormack LJ, Poutasse EF. The atrophic kidney: Its role in hypertension. *Mayo Clin Proc* 1965; 40:834–852.
17. Olin JW, Novick AC: Renovascular disease. In Young JR, Olin JW, Bartholomew JR (eds): **Peripheral Vascular Diseases**. St. Louis, MO, C.V. Mosby Co., second edition, 1996, pp 321–341.
18. Olin, JW. Evaluation of the peripheral circulation. In Izzo JL Jr, Black HR (eds): **Hypertension Primer**, Baltimore, MD, Lippincott Williams & Wilkins, second edition 1999, pp 323–326.
19. Simon N, Franklin SS, Bleifer KH, et al. Clinical characteristics of renovascular hypertension. *JAMA* 1972; 220:1209–1218.
20. Eipper DF, Gifford RW Jr, Stewart BH, et al. Abdominal bruits in renovascular hypertension. *Am J Cardiol* 1976; 37:48–52.
21. Hunt JC, Sheps SG, Harrison EG Jr, et al. Renal and renovascular hypertension. *Arch Intern Med* 1974; 133:988–999.
22. Caps MT, Zierler E, Polissar NL, et al. Risk of atrophy in kidneys with atherosclerotic renal artery stenosis. *Kid Internat* 1998; 53:735–742.
23. Textor SC, Novick AC, Tarazi RC, et al. Critical perfusion pressure for renal function in patients with bilateral atherosclerotic renal vascular disease. *Ann Intern Med* 1985; 102:308–314.
24. Jacobson HR. Ischemic renal disease: An overlooked clinical entity? *Kid Internat* 1988; 34:729–743.
25. Pickering TG, Herman L, Devereux RB, et al. Recurrent pulmonary oedema in hypertension due to bilateral renal artery stenosis: Treatment by angioplasty or surgical revascularization. *Lancet* 1988; 2:551–552.
26. Messina LM, Zelenock GB, Yao KA, et al. Renal revascularization for recurrent pulmonary edema in patients with poorly controlled hypertension and renal insufficiency: A distinct subgroup of patients with arteriosclerotic renal artery occlusive disease. *J Vasc Surg* 1992; 15:73–82.
27. Gray BH, Olin JW, Childs MB, et al. Clinical benefit of renal artery angioplasty with stenting for the control of recurrent and refractory congestive heart failure. *Circulation* 1998; 98(suppl): I-485.
28. Nally JV, Chen C, Fine E, et al. Diagnostic criteria for renal vascular hypertension with captopril renography. A consensus statement. *Am J Hyper* 1991; 4(Suppl): 749–752.
29. Olin JW, Piedmonte MR, Young JR, et al. The utility of duplex ultrasound scanning of the renal arteries for diagnosing significant renal artery stenosis. *Ann Intern Med* 1995; 122:833–838.

30. Platts AD. CT angiography with spiral angiography. In Novick A, Scoble J, Hamilton G (eds): **Renal Vascular Disease**. London, WB Saunders Co., Ltd., 1996, pp 143–149.
31. Gedroyc W. Magnetic resonance angiography of the renal arteries. In Novick A, Scoble J, Hamilton G (eds): **Renal Vascular Disease**. London, WB Saunders Co., Ltd., 1996, pp 91–106.
32. Kim D, Porter DH, Brown R, et al. Renal artery imaging: A prospective comparison of intra-arterial digital subtraction angiography with conventional angiography. *Angiology* 1991; 42:345–357.
33. Schreier DZ, Weaver FA, Frankhouse J, et al. A prospective study of carbon dioxide-digital subtraction vs standard contrast arteriography in the evaluation of renal arteries. *Arch Surg* 1996; 131:503–507.

2

Diagnosis of Renal Artery Stenosis:

What is the Optimal Diagnostic Test?

Michael R. Jaff, DO and Jeffrey W. Olin, DO

Introduction

Atherosclerosis is the most common etiology of renal artery stenosis (RAS) accounting for more than 90% of all cases. Fibromuscular dysplasia may also occur, and is found predominantly in the young patient with significant hypertension.[1] Clinical scenarios suggestive of RAS are often the most reliable indicator of the disorder. Patients with RAS may present with hypertension, azotemia or unexplained episodes of congestive heart failure or "flash" pulmonary edema.[2] In addition, the finding of discrepancy in renal size, hypertension and unexplained azotemia, or the finding of hypertension in the face of systemic atherosclerosis should prompt the clinician to search for RAS (Table 1). Early identification and treatment of patients with significant RAS is important in order to decrease associated morbidity and mortality.

There are many tests that can be used to evaluate the renal arteries. Some tests primarily provide anatomical information about the kidneys and the blood flow through the renal arteries, while others are based on the physiologic functioning of the kidney and the renin angiotensin aldosterone axis. The goal of screening is to have sufficient sensitivity and specificity to identify the patient with RAS and avoid unnecessary and costly diagnostic studies in patients

From Jaff MR (ed): *Endovascular Therapy for Atherosclerotic Renal Artery Stenosis: Present and Future*. Armonk, NY: Future Publishing Co, Inc.; ©2001.

Table 1.

Clinical Clues to Suggest the Diagnosis of Renovascular Disease.

Onset of hypertension before the age of 30 or after the age of 55
Hypertension that was well controlled and has become difficult to control
Malignant or accelerated hypertension
Resistant hypertension
Epigastric bruit (systolic/diastolic)
Atrophic kidney or discrepancy in size between the two kidneys
Azotemia while receiving angiotensin converting enzyme inhibitors or angiotensin II antag-
    onists
Azotemia in the elderly patient with atherosclerosis elsewhere
Patients with generalized atherosclerosis
Patients with unexplained congestive heart failure or "flash" pulmonary edema

who are unlikely to have the disease. While most physicians consider angiography the "gold standard" diagnostic test, it is obviously not the best screening test. The available diagnostic tests that may be used to make the diagnosis of renal artery stenosis are listed in Table 2. This chapter will focus on those tests that have sufficient sensitivity and specificity to confirm or refute the diagnosis of renal artery stenosis.

Table 2.

Diagnostic Studies to Evaluate for the Presence of Renal Artery Stenosis.

Diagnostic Study	Useful?
Intravenous pyelogram	No
Plasma renin activity	No
Captopril test	No
Renal vein renin sampling	No
Renal scintigraphy	No
Renal scintigraphy with captopril (captopril renogram)	Yes
Renal artery duplex ultrasonography	Yes
Spiral CT scanning	Yes
Magnetic resonance angiography (MRA)	Yes
Intravascular Ultrasound	Yes
CO_2 angiography	Yes
Angiography	Yes

Hypertensive Intravenous Pyelography

Intravenous pyelography (IVP) was one of the earliest tests used to diagnose RAS. The hypertensive IVP, as it was known, used criteria such as kidney length, delayed calyceal appearance of contrast, and increased renal concentration on late films to diagnose renal artery stenosis.[3] This test has fallen out of favor due to the relatively low sensitivity when compared to contrast angiography.[3,4] In the Cooperative Study of Renovascular Hypertension, 11.4% of patients with primary (essential) hypertension had a positive intravenous urogram and 17% of patients with angiographically documented significant RAS had a normal intravenous urogram.[3] A false-positive rate as high as 41% has been reported by some investigators.[3] Given the large number of more accurate studies now available to assist in making the diagnosis of RAS, the hypertensive IVP should be reviewed for its historical interest only, and should not be considered as a useful method of diagnosis for RAS.

Plasma Renin Activity and the Captopril Test

Isolated assay for plasma renin activity (PRA) has a very poor specificity for the diagnosis of RAS. It may be elevated in patients with RAS, however, a significant number of patients with essential hypertension will also have elevated PRA. In addition, patients with RAS may have low, normal, or high levels of PRA.[1,2] Patients with bilateral RAS or RAS to a solitary functioning kidney often have volume-mediated hypertension with resultant suppression of PRA.[2] In a series of 540 patients, PRA had a sensitivity of 57% and specificity of 66% in diagnosing RAS. In this series there was a false-negative rate of 43% and a false-positive rate of 34%.[5]

In an effort to improve the accuracy of PRA, the administration of an angiotensin converting enzyme inhibitor (ACEI) has been added to provide a "stimulation" test. The captopril test (as distinguished from captopril renography or scintigraphy) may serve as a physiologic marker of RAS. Plasma renin activity is measured at baseline. Captopril 50 mg is administered orally and PRA is measured 60 minutes later. Published data regarding the captopril test has demonstrated sensitivity ranging from 34%–100% with a specificity of 80%–96%.[6-9] A practical limitation of this test centers around the need to discontinue most antihypertensive medications prior to the performance of the PRA, which is often impractical. The captopril test has low accuracy in patients with renal insufficiency or bilateral RAS. This diagnostic test should not be used in current algorithms for the diagnosis of RAS.

Renal Scintigraphy

Radionuclide imaging studies can effectively evaluate renal blood flow and the excretory function of the kidney. However, the sensitivity and specificity of unstimulated renal scintigraphy is similar to that of the hypertensive IVP, and should not be used as the sole method of diagnosis in RAS.

When a baseline renal flow scan is obtained followed by a second renal flow scan obtained after the administration of the angiotensin converting enzyme inhibitor captopril, the test has excellent utility in diagnosing RAS, especially in those patients with unilateral disease.[10–12] Captopril renography involves using a glomerular radionuclide tracer and performing dynamic renal scintigraphy before and 1 hour after the oral administration of captopril 25 mg. Captopril produces an acute and reversible decrement in renal function on the ipsilateral side to the renal artery stenosis whereas renal function (glomerular filtration) will remain normal on the contralateral (nonstenotic) side.[12] The captopril renogram provides useful information regarding the size of the kidney as well as the perfusion and excretory function.

The sensitivity of captopril renography in identifying patients with renovascular disease is approximately 90% (range 83%–94%) and the specificity is approximately 93% (range of 85%–100%).[10–12] However, the sensitivity of captopril renography diminishes markedly in the presence of bilateral RAS or in patients who have significant azotemia (serum creatinine exceeding 2.5 mg/dL).[2,12]

Unfortunately, it is estimated that 50% of patients have bilateral RAS. In addition, most antihypertensive medications, including diuretics, must be discontinued for 72 hours prior to performance of captopril renal scintigraphy. Therefore, although accurate in the ideal patient (unilateral RAS with normal renal function), this is not a reliable screening test for the majority of elderly patients who may have bilateral disease and impaired renal function.

Renal Vein Renin Sampling

Renal vein renin sampling is not a useful test to screen for the presence of renal artery stenosis. This is an invasive procedure that is used in uncommon scenarios once the diagnosis of RAS has been established. For example, patients whose indication for revascularization is uncertain in the presence of RAS may benefit from renal vein renin assays to predict a beneficial response in blood pressure after angioplasty and stent implantation or surgical revascularization.[13] The patient should be off all medications that can either stimulate or suppress renin activity. Lateralizing renal vein renin ratios in a patient with a short duration of hypertension (< 5 years) predicts a high likelihood of cure of hypertension with a revascularization procedure.[14]

Duplex Ultrasonography

Duplex ultrasound, combining real-time, gray scale B-mode ultrasound, color coded imaging, and Doppler examination, has proven useful in the diagnosis of RAS. Improved commercially available equipment has led to better visualization of the renal arteries, resulting in accurate Doppler interrogation of

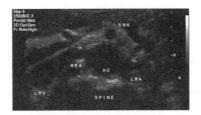

Figure 1. Gray scale ultrasound in the transverse plane demonstrating the relationship between important landmark structures. SMA = superior mesenteric artery; LRV = left renal vein; LRA = left renal artery; AO = aorta; RRA = right renal artery.

the entire renal artery (Figure 1). Duplex ultrasonography is an excellent screening test for the presence of RAS for several reasons:

1) Duplex ultrasonography provides anatomic information concerning the location of stenosis.
2) Accurate estimate of renal size is routinely obtained.
3) The test is not altered by antihypertensive medications, therefore allowing patients to continue medications throughout the test without risk of exacerbation of blood pressure.
4) There are no nephrotoxic aspects to the examination, so that it can be performed even in patients with significant azotemia
5) The test is less expensive than other tests such as spiral computed tomography (CT) scanning, magnetic resonance angiography (MRA) or angiography.[15] Sensitivity and specificity has been estimated at 75%–95% and 87%–100% respectively.[16–21]

If the ratio of the peak systolic velocity (PSV) in the renal artery to the PSV in the aorta (RAR) is 3.5 or greater, the degree of stenosis is classified between 60%–99%. If the end diastolic velocity is ≥ 150 cm/sec, this suggests a stenosis severity > 80% (Figure 2). If the RAR is < 3.5 and the PSV is < 200 cm/sec, the artery is classified as 0%–59% stenosis, and if there is an absence of flow and

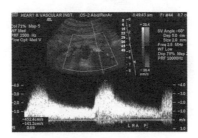

Figure 2. Color duplex ultrasound with Doppler velocity evidence of a renal artery stenosis (See Color Plate).

Table 3.

Comparison of Duplex Ultrasound with Angiography.					
Percent Stenosis by Arteriogram					
Ultrasound (%)	*0–59*	*60–79*	*80–99*	*100*	*Total*
0–59	62	0	1	1	64
60–99	1	31	67	0	99
100	0	1	1	22	24
Total	63	32	69	23	187

Sensitivity – 98%, specificity – 98%, positive predictive value – 99%, negative predictive value – 97%

From Olin JW, Piedmonte MA, Young JR, et al.[16]

a low-amplitude parenchymal signal, the artery is occluded. In one prospective study of 102 patients (187 renal arteries) comparing duplex ultrasonography to angiography,[16] the sensitivity, specificity, and predictive values were excellent for duplex scanning. The results are shown in Table 3. In addition to screening for the presence of RAS, duplex ultrasound is useful in following patients who have undergone renal artery revascularization to assess for the presence of restenosis.

The biggest criticism of renal artery duplex scanning has been the belief that results in large academic medical centers cannot be reproduced in the majority of medical centers. However, in multicenter randomized trials evaluating the safety and efficacy of various renal artery stent designs where duplex ultrasonography is used as the primary method of follow-up, after an aggressive training program by a core vascular laboratory, only 15% of examinations were unable to be completed (Jaff MR, unpublished data). A major limitation of renal artery duplex ultrasonography has been difficulty in identifying and interrogating accessory renal arteries. Hanson et al. reported a sensitivity of only 67%, but once the accessory renal artery is identified, the specificity was 100% (Figure 3).[21]

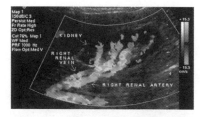

Figure 3. Renal artery duplex image obtained from the oblique (lateral decubitus) position, demonstrating the entire length of the renal artery from origin of the renal artery to the hilum of the kidney (See Color Plate).

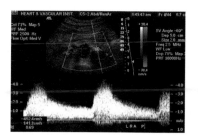

Figure 2. Color duplex ultrasound with Doppler velocity evidence of a renal artery stenosis.

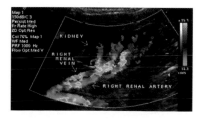

Figure 3. Renal artery duplex image obtained from the oblique (lateral decubitus) position, demonstrating the entire length of the renal artery from origin of the renal artery to the hilum of the kidney.

Magnetic Resonance Angiography

Magnetic resonance angiography is rapidly becoming the screening test of choice for RAS. There are many advantages of MRA, not the least of which is that MRA provides a visual image that is interpretable by most vascular physicians. Due to improvements in hardware and software, prior limitations of MRA such as overestimation of moderate stenoses as occlusions no longer exist in selected centers. The images obtained are reconstructed and processed to provide both two- and three-dimensional images. In addition, intravenous contrast with gadolinium and other newer MR contrast agents may overcome some of the flow dependent loss of signal and provide better images of both the main renal arteries as well as accessory renal arteries (Figure 4). The sensitivity and specificity for detecting stenosis > 60% ranges from 73%–100% and 76%–100 %, respectively.[22–26] Thorton et al.[27] recently reported sensitivity, specificity and accuracy of 100%, 98%, and 99% using a gadolinium-enhanced breath hold method.

MRA is generally well tolerated and may be performed in patients with renal insufficiency. There are limitations to the examination including poor vi-

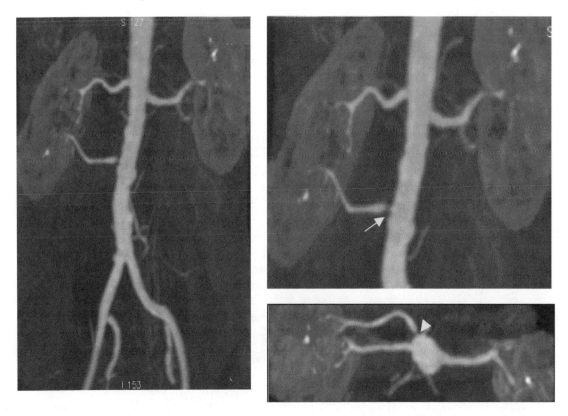

Figure 4. Magnetic resonance angiogram demonstrating stenosis of an accessory right renal artery (arrow).

sualization of the distal segment of the renal artery and assessing branch disease, especially when gadolinium is not used. Quality does vary considerably from center to center, based on available equipment and expertise in MR technology. In addition, technical considerations such as respiratory artifact, peristaltic bowel motion artifact, and claustrophobia may contribute to a nondiagnostic study. Patients with metal clips or staples, pacemakers or other metallic devices may not be candidates for examination. Economic pressures have also limited the use of MR for renal artery disease diagnosis. Presently, the Health Care Financing Administration does provide reimbursement for MRA of renal arteries unless the study is performed prior to surgical repair of an abdominal aortic aneurysm.

CT Angiography

Computed tomography angiography is performed using rapid sequence helical scanning after the administration of a bolus of intravenous iodinated contrast. The acquired images can be reformatted using several techniques to produce two- or three-dimensional reconstructions, resulting in accurate demonstration of the renal arteries. Several series have reported sensitivity for diagnosing RAS using CT angiography as 59%–92 %, with specificity as 82%–98 %.[28–31] Prokop[32] has provided an excellent review of the technical aspects of CT angiography and suggests that in optimal situations, the sensitivity and specificity of the test is between 90%–98% and the negative predictive value is greater than 95%.[32,33] Thus a normal CT angiogram essentially rules out RAS. In addition, the spiral CT scan also allows identification of the aorta, kidneys, adrenal glands and other structures, providing additional data that other noninvasive imaging studies of the renal arteries may not provide. Similar to MRA and contrast angiography, CT angiography has the ability to identify accessory renal arteries. Unlike MRA, the examination is not limited by metallic devices or pacemakers and the claustrophobic patient usually finds the exam tolerable.

This examination requires a large contrast load, thereby making this a less useful tool in patients with pre-existing azotemia. In addition, some patients may not be capable of performing the prolonged breath hold required to minimize the respiratory artifact. Occasionally, opacification of the renal veins may obscure the renal arteries or accessory renal arteries and limit the diagnostic ability of the examination. Similar to MRA, postprocessing software varies between institutions, resulting in differing levels of accuracy.[31–33]

Arteriography

Arteriography remains the gold standard for the diagnosis of RAS. If the clinical suspicion for RAS is high, even with negative noninvasive studies, the patient should undergo arteriography especially if intervention will be offered in the face of positive results.

Figure 5 shows a diagnostic algorithm that may be of help in planning diagnostic strategies for the diagnosis of RAS. The inclusion of renal duplex scan-

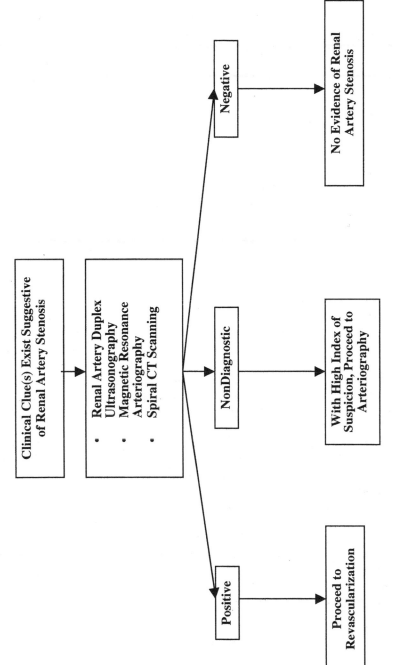

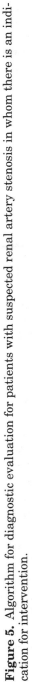

Figure 5. Algorithm for diagnostic evaluation for patients with suspected renal artery stenosis in whom there is an indication for intervention.

ning as a first line screening test reflects consideration of economic issues and the fact that duplex ultrasonography is as effective a screening method as MRA in centers with interest and expertise in this technique.

Conclusion

Duplex ultrasonography, MRA, and CT angiography must be viewed as the primary screening tests for the diagnosis of RAS. When positive, these tests can reliably confirm the diagnosis of RAS. Unfortunately, none of the available screening modalities has the ability to predict which patients will benefit from surgical or endovascular revascularization. It is for this reason that an appropriate clinical evaluation, with appreciation of clinical clues to the diagnosis of RAS, be performed prior to any testing. Since many of the commonly used noninvasive tests have considerable technical limitations, not all centers will have the equipment and expertise to perform reliable noninvasive testing. Physicians should use the diagnostic test that is most accurate and safe, and will likely vary from center to center and physician to physician.

References

1. Canzanello VJ, Textor SC. Noninvasive diagnosis of renovascular disease. *Mayo Clin Proc* 1994; 69:1172–1181.
2. Olin JW, Novick AC. Renovascular disease. In Young JR, Olin JW, Bartholomew JR (eds). Peripheral Vascular Diseases. St. Louis, CV Mosby Co, second edition, 1996.
3. Bookstein JJ, Abrams HL, Buenger RE, et al. Radiologic aspects of renovascular hypertension. Part 2. The role of urography in unilateral renovascular disease. *JAMA* 1972; 220(9): 1225–1230.
4. Bookstein JJ, Abrams HL, Buenger RE, et al. Radiologic aspects of renovascular hypertension. Part 1. Aims and methods of the radiology study group. *JAMA* 1972; 220(9)1218–1224.
5. Maxwell MH, Rudnick MR, Waks AU. New approaches to the diagnosis of renovascular hypertension. *Adv Nephrol Necker Hosp* 1985; 14:285–304.
6. Elliott WJ, Martin WB, Murphy MB. Comparison of two noninvasive screening tests for renovascular hypertension. *Arch Intern Med* 1993; 153:755–764.
7. Frederickson ED, Wilcox CS, Bucci CM, et al. A prospective evaluation of a simplified captopril test for the detection of renovascular hypertension. *Arch Intern Med* 1990; 150:569–572.
8. Muller FB, Sealey JE, Case DB, et al. The captopril test for identifying renovascular disease in hypertensive patients. *Am J Med* 1986; 80:633–644.
9. Postma CT, van der Steen PHM, Hoefnagels WHL, et al. The captopril test in the detection of renovascular disease in hypertensive patients. *Arch Intern Med* 1990; 150:625–628.
10. Mann SJ, Pickering TG, Sos TA, et al. Captopril renography in the diagnosis of renal artery stenosis: Accuracy and limitations. *Am J Med* 1991; 90:30–40.
11. Taylor AT Jr, Fletcher JW, Nally JV Jr, et al. Procedure guideline for diagnosis of renovascular hypertension. Society of Nuclear Medicine. *J Nucl Med* 1998; 39:1297–1302.
12. Nally JV Jr, Black HR. State-of-the-art review: Captopril renography–pathophysiological considerations and clinical observations. *Semin Nucl Med* 1992; 22:85–97.
13. Maxwell MH, Marks LS, Lupu AN, et al. Predictive value of renin determinations in renal artery stenosis. *JAMA* 1977; 238:2617–2620.
14. Hughes JS, Dove HG, Gifford RW Jr, et al. Duration of blood pressure elevation in

accurately predicting surgical cure of renovascular hypertension. *Am Heart J* 1981; 101:408–413.

15. Olin JW. Role of duplex ultrasonography in screening for significant renal artery disease. *Urol Clin N Am* 1994; 21:215–226.
16. Olin JW, Piedmonte MR, Young JR, et al. The utility of duplex ultrasound scanning of the renal arteries for diagnosing significant renal artery stenosis. *Ann Intern Med* 1995; 122:833–838.
17. Hoffman U, Edwards JM, Carter S, et al. Role of duplex scanning for the detection of atherosclerotic renal artery disease. *Kid Internat* 1991; 39:1232–1239.
18. Mollo M, Pelet V, Mouawad J, et al. Evaluation of colour duplex ultrasound scanning in diagnosis of renal artery stenosis, compared to angiography: A prospective study on 53 patients. *Eur J Vasc Endovasc Surg* 1997; 14:305–309.
19. Zoller WG, Hermans H, Bogner JR, et al. Duplex sonography in the diagnosis of renovascular hypertension. *Klin Wochenschr* 1990; 68:830–834.
20. Miralles M, Santiso A, Gimenez A, et al. Renal duplex scanning: Correlation with angiography and isotopic renography. *Eur J Vasc Surg* 1993; 7:188–194.
21. Hansen KJ, Tribble RW, Reavis SW, et al. Renal duplex sonography: Evaluation of clinical utility. *J Vasc Surg* 1990; 12:227–236.
22. Leung DA, Hoffman U, Pfammatter T, et al. Magnetic resonance angiography versus duplex sonography for diagnosing renovascular disease. *Hypertension* 1999; 33:726–731.
23. Borrello JA, Li D, Vesely TM, et al. Renal arteries: Clinical comparison of three-dimensional time-of-flight MR angiographic sequences and radiographic angiography. *Radiology* 1995; 197:793–799.
24. Hertz SM, Holland GA, Baum RA, et al. Evaluation of renal artery stenosis by magnetic resonance angiography. *Am J Surg* 1994; 168:140–143.
25. Loubeyre P, Revel D, Garcia P, et al. Screening patients for renal artery stenosis: Value of three-dimensional time-of-flight MR angiography. *Am J Roentgenol* 1994; 162:847–852.
26. Kent KC, Edelman RR, Kim D, et al. Magnetic resonance imaging: A reliable test for the evaluation of proximal atherosclerotic renal arterial stenosis. *J Vasc Surg* 1991; 13:311–318.
27. Thornton MJ, Thornton F, O'Callaghan J, et al. Evaluation of dynamic gadolinium-enhanced breath-hold MR angiography in the diagnosis of renal artery stenosis. *Am J Roentgenol* 1999; 173:1279–1283.
28. Rubin GD, Dake MD, Napel S, et al. Spiral CT of renal artery stenosis: Comparison of three-dimensional rendering techniques. *Radiology* 1994; 190:181–189.
29. Elkohen M, Beregi JP, Deklunder G, et al. A prospective study of helical computed tomography angiography versus angiography for the detection of renal artery stenosis in hypertensive patients. *J Hypertension* 1996; 14:525–528.
30. Johnson PT, Halpern EJ, Kuszyk BS, et al. Renal artery stenosis: CT angiography-comparison of real-time volume-rendering and maximal intensity projection algorithms. Radiology 1999; 211:337–343.
31. Galanski M, Prokop M, Chavan A, et al. Renal artery stenoses: Spiral CT angiography. *Radiology* 1993; 189:185–192.
32. Prokop M. Protocols and future directions in imaging of renal artery stenosis: CT angiography. *J Comput Assist Tomogr* 1999; 23 (Suppl 1): S101-S110.
33. Wittenberg G, Kenn W, Tschammler A, et al. Spiral CT angiography of the renal arteries: Comparison with angiography. *Eur Radiol* 1999:9: 546–51.

3

The Natural History of Atherosclerotic Renal Artery Stenosis:

Is This Truly a Progressive Disorder?

DE Strandness Jr., MD, D Med (Hon)

Introduction

It was the classic contributions of Goldblatt in the 1930s that established the role of renal artery stenosis (RAS) in the development of hypertension.[1] The true incidence of RAS has been difficult to estimate due to our lack of simple, direct methods of detecting its presence.[2] It was the problem of hypertension that occupied most of our attention until we became aware of the potential contribution of renal artery disease to the development of ischemic renal failure. Since the hypertension secondary to RAS was potentially curable, surgery was frequently carried out to relieve the narrowing. However, even though RAS was corrected, the hypertension was often not cured. Thus, it became clear that there were other factors that contributed to the continued problem of blood pressure control.

While there is still a great deal of interest in the issue of blood pressure control, the potential role for the renal artery disease in the development of ischemic renal failure has become an important issue.[3] Since this should only occur with high grade lesions, it will be important to determine when and at what rate renal artery stenoses progress to the level where renal failure might occur.[4]

From Jaff MR (ed): *Endovascular Therapy for Atherosclerotic Renal Artery Stenosis: Present and Future*. Armonk, NY: Future Publishing Co, Inc.; ©2001.

In order to sort out these issues it is necessary to study the individual elements of this complex problem that may be contributing to the development of both hypertension and ischemic renal failure. We believe that ultrasonic duplex scanning properly done can be used for this purpose.[5-7] This chapter describes our results in a prospective long-term follow-up study of atherosclerotic RAS.

Materials and Methods

In 1990 a prospective study of the natural history of RAS was started. When the first phase of this study was completed in 1997, a total of 220 subjects had been recruited.[8-11] The patients included in the study had to have at least one of the renal arteries involved. The indications for screening that led to the discovery of the renal lesions were hypertension, renal insufficiency or both. No patients who were considered candidates for some form of intervention were recruited. Once enrolled in the study, the therapy for the patient was provided by the referring physician and not by the research team. After each visit, a letter was sent to the physician indicating the findings but without recommendations as to treatment. Only those patients who had been followed a minimum of 3 months were included in the final analysis.

The patients (sides) who were excluded from this analysis were as follows:

(1) Twenty-one renal arteries that were found to be occluded at the time of the initial evaluation.
(2) One patient had a congenitally absent kidney with the contralateral side having an incomplete duplex evaluation.
(3) We excluded all kidneys less than 8.5 cms in length (11). These included those with renal artery occlusion whose mean kidney length at time of entry into the study was 7.2 ± 1.3 cm. If cysts were found that were between 2 and 4 cms in diameter, the involved kidney was not excluded unless they involved the poles of the kidney, making an estimate of renal length difficult.
(4) This left 170 subjects—295 renal arteries for the final analysis.
(5) After the initial evaluation, each patient was restudied every six months. In those cases where some form of intervention was performed during follow-up, all subsequent examinations were excluded from the analysis.

The detection and classification of the degree of narrowing was based upon the duplex findings shown in Table 1. It is not the purpose of this chapter to review the accuracy of the method.[5-7] This has been done showing a sensitivity

Table 1.

Comparison of Duplex versus Arteriography for the Detection of a > 60% Stenosis.

	Arteriography			
Duplex	< 60% Stenosis	> 60% Stenosis	Occluded	Total
RAR < 3.5	15	3	1	19
RAR > 3.5	11	45	0	56
Occluded	0	0	10	10
Total	26	48	11	

Sensitivity 92%, Specificity 58%, accuracy 81%, Kappa statistic 0.66. The lower specificity was due to difference as to whether the lesion was greater or less than 60%, RAR = renal aortic ratio.

and specificity in excess of 90%. The sources of these data are to be found in the references.[12]

Outcome Variables

While control of blood pressure is an extremely important variable, we were interested in examining those factors that appear to be related to the loss of renal mass (length) and progression of the RAS.[13] These two endpoints require different types of analysis which are as follows:

(1) Renal atrophy was defined as a loss of renal length. This required measurement of kidney length at the time of each visit. The threshold of measurement for documenting atrophy was placed at a 1 cm loss in length. We used this since our studies showed that the variability between observations in estimating renal length was 0.55 cm. The standard deviation of all points about the regression line was 0.39 cms which yielded a between observation variability of 0.55 cm ($0.39 \times 2_{\frac{1}{2}}$). Hence a reduction of 1 cm or more in length appeared to be unlikely in the absence of a true change in size.[3]

(2) Renal artery disease progression. If the patient moved from one of our diagnostic groups to the next higher during follow-up they were listed as "progressors."
   a. Normal to < 60%
   b. < 60% to > 60%
   c. < 60%, > 60%, > 60% to total occlusion

(3) One of the problems was to define what is meant by progression within a category. For example, if a stenosis with a resultant diameter reduction were to get worse, how could we detect it? As noted above, we can document progression by category (< 60% to > 60%, and total occlusion), but what about the progression rate within the 60%–99% category? Since this is the most severe disease and the one that most likely contributes to loss of renal mass, this is the one category where progression might be critically important. For example, if the lesion were to move from a 70% to a 99% stenosis this could be consistent with the development of progressive renal ischemia. We postulated that a change between visits in the peak systolic velocity at the site of stenosis of greater than 100 cms/sec was likely to be associated with true progression. As noted in our 1998 report we used this value to signify true progression for those lesions in the 60%–99% category.[9]

Results

The baseline characteristics of the kidneys in the study population and the relationship with atrophy are shown in Table 2. A decrease of renal length of >1 cm was found in 33 of the 204 kidneys (16.2%).[10] The baseline lengths found at entry are similar to what one would expect in an age and sex matched population without RAS. The Cumulative Incidence of renal atrophy based upon the initial disease classification is as follows:

(1) Atrophy occurred in 5.5% of kidneys with no RAS at baseline.
(2) It was 11.5% for those who started with a < 60% stenosis.
(3) It was 20.8% in those with a ≥ 60% diameter stenosis.

Table 2.

Characteristics at Time of Entry into the Study.

Characteristic	Statistic	Value	Number of kidneys
Number of Kidneys			204
Length of follow-up	mean (range)	33 (5–72) months	204
Renal Length	mean (range)	10.8 (8.8–14.5) cms	204
Stenosis severity			
PSV cm/sec	mean ± SD	296 ± 141	
RAR	mean ± SD	4.0 ± 2.0	204
Disease Class			
Normal	percent	21%	204
< 60%	percent	30%	204
≥ 60%	percent	49%	204
Renal cortical blood flow			
CPSV cm/sec	mean ± SD	20.5 ± 7.7	204
CEDV	mean ± SD	60 ± 2.5	204

PSV – Peak Systolic Velocity, CPSV – cortical peak systolic velocity, CEDV – cortical end diastolic velocity, RAR = renal aortic ratio.

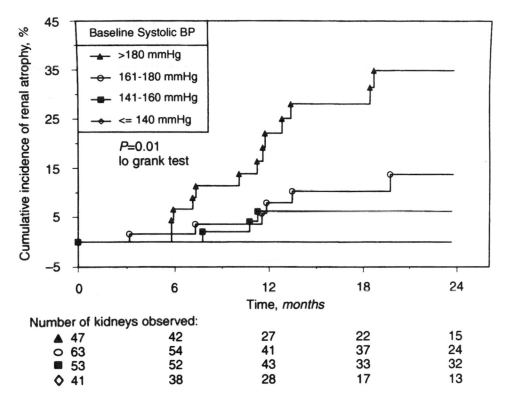

Number of kidneys observed:

▲ 47	42	27	22	15
○ 63	54	41	37	24
■ 53	52	43	33	32
◇ 41	38	28	17	13

Figure 1. Cumulative incidence of renal atrophy stratified according to baseline systolic blood pressure. The standard error is < 10% for all plots. (From Caps MT, Zierler RE, Polissar NL, et al. Risk of atrophy in kidneys with atherosclerotic renal artery stenosis. *Kid Internat* 1998;53:735–742. By Permission)

Of great importance is to determine those factors that might be contributing to the loss of renal mass. As a part of our evaluation, we also examined a variety of risk factors that might be of importance. One of the remarkable findings was the relationship between data collected at the time of the initial visit and long-term outcome. A Cox proportional hazards analysis between the baseline factors and risk of atrophy are shown in Table 3. The

Table 3.

Cox Stepwise Hazards Analysis between Baseline Risk Factors for Renal Artery Disease Progression.

Factor	RR	95% CI	P
sbp ± 160 mmHg	2.1	1.2–3.5	0.006
Diabetes mellitus	2.0	1.2–2.3	0.009
High grade ipsilateral stenosis	1.9	1.2–3.0	0.004
High grade contralateral stenosis	1.7	1.0, 2.8	0.04

RR = relative risk, high grade ± 60% stenosis.

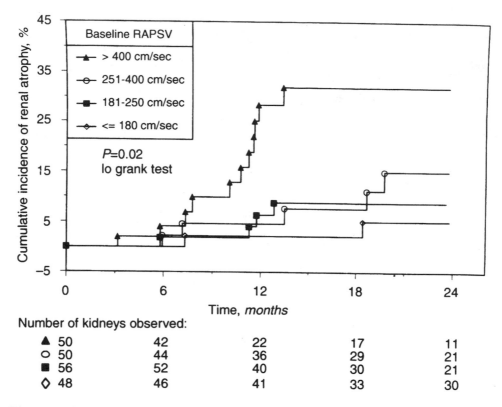

Figure 2. Cumulative incidence of renal atrophy stratified by the baseline peak systolic velocity at the site of the stenosis at the time of entry. The standard error is < 10% for all plots. (From Caps MT, Zierler RE, Polissar NL, et al. Risk of atrophy in kidneys with atherosclerotic renal artery stenosis. *Kid Internat* 1998;53:735–742. By permission.)

graphic representations of these factors and their influence are shown in Figures 1–3.

(1) Systolic blood pressure at entry (Figure 1).
(2) Baseline peak systolic velocity at the site of the stenosis (Figure 2).
(3) Baseline cortical end diastolic velocity (Figure 3).

Renal Artery Disease Progression

For this evaluation, we included 295 kidneys in 170 patients who were studied for a mean of 33 months. The three year cumulative incidence of renal artery disease progression was 18%, 28%, and 49% respectively for those kidneys whose renal arteries were classified at the time of entry to be normal, < 60% stenosis, or > 60% stenosis. Progression to renal artery occlusion occurred in < 10% of the kidneys with a < or > 60% stenosis at entry. There was not a

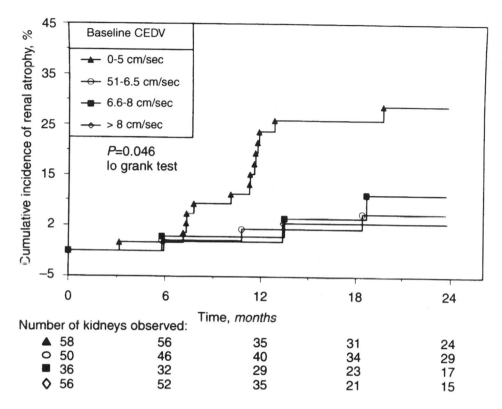

Figure 3. Cumulative incidence of renal atrophy based upon the cortical end-diastolic velocity at the time of entry. The standard error is < 10% for all plots. (From Caps MT, Zierler RE, Polissar NL, et al. Risk of atrophy in kidneys with atherosclerotic renal artery stenosis. *Kid Internat* 1998;53:735–742. By permission.)

single instance of progression to occlusion when the artery was seen to be normal at the time of entry.

When a stepwise Cox proportional hazards analysis was considered, it was apparent that there were four factors that appeared to be related to progression of the renal artery lesion.[1] (Table 4).

Table 4.

Cox Stepwise Hazard Analysis for Renal Atrophy.

Factor	RR	95% CI	P
systolic blood pressure, per 20 mmHg increase	2.1	1.3–3.5	< 0.001
severity of renal artery stenosis, per 100 cm/sec increase	1.5	1.2–1.9	< 0.001
cortical peak systolic velocity, per 5 cm/sec decrease	1.7	1.0–1.7	< 0.05
cortical end diastolic velocity, per 2 cm/sec decrease	2.1	1.3–3.6	< 0.01

RR = relative risk, CI = confidence intervals.

Discussion

It is apparent to most workers in this field that the true prevalence of RAS has been greatly underestimated. This has in large part been due to the fact that there have not been direct and accurate methods, short of arteriography, to detect the lesion. The situation with regard to the role of atherosclerotic RAS has been greatly complicated by the nearly simultaneous development of parenchymal vascular disease.[14] This was also predicted by Goldblatt, who showed that the kidney opposite a site of RAS could develop arteriolar nephrosclerosis that would possibly make the treatment of the hypertension more difficult. This would appear to be a fact if one looks at the success/failure for direct intervention in terms of blood pressure control alone. It is generally accepted that actual "cure" of the hypertension occurs in less than 10% of cases where this has been done. This is in sharp contrast to the patients (largely women) who develop fibromuscular dysplasia (FMD) hypertension.[15,16] This entity, which can also lead to very severe narrowing of the renal artery, does not appear to develop the parenchymal lesions seen with atherosclerosis. It is my belief that this is why they do much better with intervention be it surgery or angioplasty for the treatment of hypertension. In addition, it is very rare for any patient with FMD to develop chronic renal failure.

The one area that has in recent years received the greatest attention is the problem of ischemic renal failure and its possible prevention by identifying and treating patients with bilateral RAS. It would appear that this may well be the point at which to examine patients who are thought to be at risk for the development of RAS and over time renal failure. The issue of screening is not within the scope of this chapter, so it will be confined to the changes that the author believes can be discovered and documented by duplex scanning.

Like many ultrasound methods, their introduction are usually met by two concerns – the test is too technologist-dependent and secondly, it is too time consuming. These complaints are still heard in some circles about renal duplex studies but these are slowly disappearing as experience in good laboratories is accumulated and published. Before considering the issues of progression, I would like to summarize our current thinking about some issues that are germane to the entire effort:

(1) It is accurate for detecting RAS.
(2) It is as accurate as arteriography for the detection of hemodynamically significant stenoses.
(3) Kidney length can be measured with a reasonable level of variability.
(4) The renal duplex study can be repeated in order to document the stability of the detected lesion(s) in the renal artery.
(5) Kidney length as a surrogate marker for renal atrophy can be measured on a repetitive basis.
(6) This method can be used to document the results of either angioplasty

with or without stenting to document the success/failure of the procedure.

(7) The method can be applied after renal artery reconstruction by surgical means to document the outcome.

It would be ideal if we could combine the use of duplex scanning with some method to document the effect of the RAS on individual kidney glomerular filtration rate (GFR). At the moment this is not practical clinically so we are forced to make some assumptions which intuitively seem to make sense. The first is that the loss of renal length is bad for the kidney and leads to loss of nephrons and if this occurs bilaterally, will lead to renal failure.

In the studies looking at the issue of loss of renal mass over time, we did see a steady rise in the levels of serum creatinine.[10] In fact, it appeared that 10% of our population would satisfy the diagnosis of ischemic renal failure. In addition, we noted that this was most likely to occur in the patients with the tighter degrees of RAS (> 60%). In addition, it appeared that the progression from a < 60% to a > 60% stenosis was what occurred in those patients where a loss of renal mass was observed.

Where are we today in this field with regard to diagnosis and therapy? My own views on this subject have been arrived at because of the studies covered in this chapter along with an appreciation of where we stand at the moment from a therapeutic standpoint. I can make the following observations that are based in large part on observed facts but to some degree on what this might mean from a therapeutic standpoint.

(1) The diagnosis of RAS is available if one is willing to look.
(2) We have come to appreciate the fact that loss of renal mass is a consequence of renal artery stenosis that is high grade and progressive over time.
(3) The resistance offered to flow by examining the cortical end-diastolic to peak systolic velocity ratio (EDR) is an area where much more work needs to be done. It is our belief that this ratio is a reflection of the resistance offered by the microvascular bed within the kidney.[17] The normal EDR should be > 0.35. Frauchiger et al. examined the relationship between EDR and the response to renal artery interventions.[15] In this very preliminary study, an EDR of < 0.3 correlated well with a failure of endovascular intervention while values above 0.3 were not predictive of outcome. It was interesting to note that patients with FMD had normal EDRs and this could well explain their more favorable response to therapy.[15,16]

References

1. Goldblatt H, Lynch J, Hanzel RF, et al. Studies on experimental hypertension. The production of persistent elevation of systolic blood pressure by means of renal ischemia. *J Exp Medicine* 1934; 59:347–379.
2. Gifford RW. Epidemiology and clinical manifestations of renovascular hyperten-

sion. In Stanley J, Stanley JECFWJ, (eds): **Renovascular Hypertension**. Philadelphia: W.B. Saunders Co., 1984 pp 77–99.

3. Isaacson JA, Zierler RE, Bergelin RO, et al. A method for minimizing variability in kidney length measurements during renal artery duplex scanning. *J Vasc Techn* 1993.

4. Tullis MJ, Zierler RE, Glickerman DJ, et al. Results of percutaneous transluminal angioplasty for atherosclerotic renal artery stenosis: A follow-up study with duplex ultrasonography. *J Vasc Surg* 1997; 25(1): 46–54.

5. Hoffman U, Edwards JM, Carter S, et al. Role of duplex scanning for the detection of athrosclerotic renal artery disease. *Kidn Int* 1991; 39:1232–1239.

6. Olin JW, Piedmonte MR, Young JR, et al. The utility of duplex ultrasound scanning of the renal arteries for diagnosing significant renal artery stenosis. *Ann Internal Medicine* 1995; 122:833–838.

7. Taylor DC, Kettler MD, Moneta GL, et al. Duplex ultrasound in the diagnosis of renal artery stenosis: A prospective evaluation. *J Vasc Surg* 1988; 7:363–369.

8. Zierler RE, Isaacson JA, Bergelin RO, et al. Natural history of renal artery stenosis: A prospective study with duplex ultrasound. *J Vasc Surg* 1994; 19:250–258.

9. Caps MT. Prospective study of atherosclerotic disease progression in the renal artery. Circulation 1998; 2866–2872. 1–22–0298.

10. Caps MT, Zierler RE, Polissar NL, et al. Risk of atrophy in kidneys with atherosclerotic renal artery stenosis. *Kidn Int* 1998; 53(3): 735–742.

11. Taylor DC, Moneta GL, Strandness DE, Jr. Follow-up of renal artery stenosis by duplex ultrasound. *J Vasc Surg* 1989; 9:410–415.

12. Hoffmann U, Edwards JM, Carter S, et al. Role of duplex scanning for the detection of atherosclerotic renal artery disease. *Kidn Int* 1991; 39(6): 1232–1239.

13. Guzman RP, Zierler RE, Isaacson JA, et al. Renal atrophy and arterial stenosis: A prospective study with duplex ultrasound. *Hypertension* 1994; 23:346–350.

14. Tullis MJ, Zierler RE, Caps MT, et al. Clinical evidence of contralateral renal parenchymal injury in patients with unilateral atherosclerotic renal artery stenosis. *Ann Vasc Surg* 1998; 12(2): 122–127.

15. Frauchiger B, Zierler R, Bergelin RO, et al. Prognostic significance of intrarenal resistance indices in patients with renal artery interventions: A preliminary duplex sonographic study. *Cardiovasc Surg* 1996; 4(3): 324–330.

16. Edwards JM. A preliminary study of the role of duplex scanning in defining the adequacy of treatment of patients with renal artery fibromuscular dysplasia. *J Vasc Surg* 1992; 15:604–609.

17. Norris DS. Noninvasive evaluation of renal artery stenosis and renovascular resistance: Experimental and clinical studies. *J Vasc Surg* 1984; 1:192–201.

4

Surgical Revascularization of Atherosclerotic Renal Artery Disease:

Results, Benefits, and Limitations

James M. Wong, MD, Timothy C. Oskin, MD, and Kimberley J. Hansen, MD

Introduction

The introduction of new, more potent antihypertensive agents and percutaneous endovascular techniques has changed many attitudes regarding surgical intervention for renovascular disease.[1] Many physicians appear to limit surgical intervention to severe hypertension despite maximal medical therapy, to failures or disease patterns not amenable to percutaneous transluminal renal artery angioplasty (PTRA) or to renovascular disease associated with excretory renal insufficiency (i.e., *ischemic nephropathy*). Consequently, our center's patient population is characterized by renal artery atherosclerosis (85%) superimposed on diffuse extrarenal atherosclerotic disease (95%). Among 534 patients treated over the past ten years, 80% of patients had at least mild renal insufficiency. Bilateral renal artery disease was found in 60% of patients, while 40% required simultaneous aortic reconstruction for clinically significant occlusive or aneurysmal disease.[2]

From Jaff MR (ed): *Endovascular Therapy for Atherosclerotic Renal Artery Stenosis: Present and Future.* Armonk, NY: Future Publishing Co, Inc.; ©2001.

Although a number of operative methods have been used to correct renal artery disease, no single technique provides the best method of repair for all renovascular lesions. Optimal methods of renal reconstruction vary with the patient, the type and pattern of renal artery disease, and the clinical significance of associated aortic lesions. This review examines the indications, results, benefits, and limitations of operative management of atherosclerotic renovascular disease.

Prevalence, Evaluation and Diagnosis

Renovascular disease is thought to account for approximately 3% of hypertension within the general population. Although its prevalence in patients with mild hypertension (diastolic blood pressure < 95 mmHg) is low, renovascular disease is a frequent cause of hypertension in patients with severe hypertension, particularly at the extremes of age. A review of 74 consecutive children evaluated for hypertension over a 5-year period showed that 78% of the children less than 5 years of age had a correctable renovascular cause.[3] After childhood, the elderly comprise the age group that has the next highest probability of having renovascular hypertension. In the 1996 academic year, the authors' center screened 629 hypertensive individuals for renovascular disease. Among patients 60 years of age and greater with diastolic blood pressure greater than or equal to 110 mmHg, 52% had significant renal artery stenosis or occlusion. When associated with an elevated serum creatinine (SCr), the prevalence increased to 71% with half of these patients demonstrating bilateral renal artery disease (unpublished data).

These data suggest the probability of finding clinically significant renal artery disease correlates with the patient's age, the severity of hypertension, and the presence and severity of renal insufficiency. With this in mind, the authors' center evaluates all persons with severe hypertension for renovascular disease; particularly children and the elderly, especially when severe hypertension is found in combination with excretory renal insufficiency.

A noninvasive screening test that accurately identifies renal artery disease in all individuals does not yet exist.[4] Currently available tests can be broadly characterized as functional or anatomic. With the exception of captopril renography, studies that rely on activation of the renin-angiotensin axis have been associated with an unacceptable rate of false negative results. Current isotope renography utilizes a variety of radiopharmaceuticals before and after exercise or converting enzyme inhibition, however, the methods used and the criteria for interpretation are continuously modified in an effort to improve the sensitivity and specificity.[5] Consequently, the authors have emphasized direct screening methods.[6] Our center utilizes renal duplex sonography as the preliminary study of choice for both renovascular hypertension and ischemic nephropathy. Through continued improvements in software and probe design, renal duplex has proven an accurate method to identify hemodynamically-significant renal artery occlusive disease with a 93% sensitivity, 98% specificity, and 96% overall accuracy.[7] The examination poses no risk to residual excretory renal function and overall accuracy is not affected by concomitant aortoiliac disease. In addition, preparation is minimal (an overnight fast) and there is no need to alter antihypertensive medications.

These results suggest that a negative renal duplex effectively excludes ischemic nephropathy, since the primary consideration is global renal ischemia based on main renal artery disease. However, when renal duplex is used to screen for renovascular hypertension, multiple or polar renal arteries and their associated disease pose a potential limitation. Despite enhanced recognition of multiple arteries provided by Doppler color-flow, only 40% of these accessory renal vessels are currently identified. Disease associated with polar vessels is particularly important when children and young adults are considered. Accordingly, the authors' group proceeds with conventional angiography in these patients when hypertension is severe or poorly controlled despite a negative duplex result.

When a unilateral renal artery lesion is confirmed by angiography, its functional significance should be defined. Both renal vein renin assays (RVRAs) and split renal function studies have proven valuable in assessing the functional significance of renovascular disease. Renal vein renin assays should demonstrate a ratio of renin activity exceeding 1.5:1.0 between involved and uninvolved sides before a presumptive diagnosis of renovascular hypertension is established. Unfortunately, neither functional study has great value when severe bilateral disease or disease to a solitary kidney is present. Therefore, the decision for empiric intervention is based on the severity of the renal artery lesions, the severity of hypertension and the degree of associated renal insufficiency. In this latter instance, issues determining recovery of excretory renal function remain ill-defined. Our center's experience with over 210 patients with severe hypertension and preoperative serum creatinine ≥ 1.8 mg/dL has demonstrated a significant association between an improved renal function response after operative intervention and the site of renal artery disease, the extent of renovascular repair, and the rate of decline in preoperative renal function.[1,8–10] Global renal disease submitted to complete renal artery repair after rapid decline in excretory renal function is associated with the best opportunity for recovery of renal function.[8,9]

Management Options

In recent years, optimal management of renal artery disease has become increasingly controversial. Advocates of medical management, PTRA, or operative management, cite selective clinical data to support their view. A majority of the medical community evaluate patients for renovascular disease only when medications are not tolerated or hypertension remains severe and uncontrolled. The study by Hunt and Strong remains the most informative study available to assess the comparative value of medical therapy and operation.[11] In their nonrandomized study, the results of operative treatment in 100 patients was compared with the results of drug therapy in 114 similar patients. After 7 to 14 years of follow-up, 84% of the operated group were alive as compared to 66% in the drug therapy group. Of the 84 patients alive in the operated group, 93% were cured or significantly improved, compared with 16 (21%) of the patients alive in the drug therapy group. Compared with surgical management, death during follow-up was twice as common in the medically treated group. Antihypertensive agents in current use provide improved blood pressure control compared with this earlier era. However, additional data regarding medical therapy for renovascular hypertension suggests that decrease in kidney size and renal function occur despite satisfactory blood pressure control.[12]

The detrimental changes that occur during medical therapy alone combined with the excellent contemporary results of operative management argue for an aggressive attitude toward renal artery intervention when renovascular hypertension is present.[1] The authors' indications for operation include all patients with severe, difficult-to-control hypertension. This includes patients with complicating factors such as branch lesions and extrarenal vascular disease and patients with associated cardiovascular disease that would be improved by blood pressure reduction. Moreover, young patients whose hypertension is moderate, who have no associated end-organ disease, and who have an easily correctable atherosclerotic or fibromuscular dysplasia (FMD) main renal artery stenosis are also candidates for intervention. The chance for cure of moderate hypertension is quite good in such patients and it remains to be proven that medical control is ever as good as the cure of hypertension. In fact, it is plausible that reduction in perfusion pressure across the stenosis by successful drug therapy may accelerate decreased renal function by further reducing glomerular pressure. Finally, no evidence exists that age, type of lesion (whether atherosclerotic or FMD), duration of hypertension, or presence of bilateral lesions has utility to estimate operative risk or of the likelihood of successful operative management. The presence or absence of these factors should not be used as determinants of management.

Percutaneous Transluminal Angioplasty with and without Stenting

Experience with the liberal use of PTRA has helped to clarify its role as a therapeutic option in the treatment of renovascular hypertension. Accumulated data argue for its selective application. In this regard, PTRA of nonostial atherosclerotic lesions and medial fibroplasia of the main renal artery yields blood pressure results comparable to the results of operative repair. In contrast, suboptimal lesions for PTRA include congenital lesions, fibrodysplastic lesions involving renal artery branches, ostial atherosclerotic lesions and renal artery occlusions. In each instance, these lesions are associated with inferior results and increased risk of complications.

A review of published reports over the past 10 years documenting blood pressure and renal function after PTRA for atherosclerotic renovascular disease reveals that 70% of patients experienced a beneficial blood pressure response (Table 1).[13–22] However, only 35% of patients with pre-existing renal insufficiency experienced improved excretory renal function while 53% remained

Table 1.

Results after PTRA for Atherosclerotic Renal Artery Stenosis.

Reference	Patients (n)	Technical Success (%)	Patients with Renal Dysfunction (n)	Function Response after Angioplasty (%)			HTN Response after Angioplasty (%)			Reste-nosis (%)	Major Compli-cations (%)	Mortality (%)
				Improved	Unchanged	Worsened	Cured	Improved	Failed			
Canzanello VJ (1989)[13]	100	73%	66	52% (36%)		48% (64%)	59% (43%)		41% (57%)	19%	20%	2.0%
Klinge J (1989)[14]	134	78%	n/r	n/r	n/r	n/r	11%	78%	11%	20%	12%	0.5%
Baert AL (1990)[15]	165	83%	n/r	n/r	n/r		32% (24%)	36% (28%)	32% (48%)	10%	11%	0%
Tykarski A (1993)[16]	26	79%	16	69%	31%	0%	45% (35%)	35% (27%)	20% (38%)	10%	8%	0%
Weibull H (1993)[17]	29	83%	n/r	21%	75%	4%	13% (10%)	71% (59%)	16% (31%)	25%	17%	0%
Losinno F (1994)[18]	153	95%	59	27%	67%	6%	12%	51%	37%	n/r	8%	0%
Rodriguez-Perez JC (1994)[19]	37	78%	n/r	no change in mean SCr			3%	80%	17%	10%	8%	n/r??
Bonelli FS (1995)[20]	190	82%	n/r	no change in mean SCr			8%	62%	30%	10%	23%	3.7%
Hoffman O (1998)[21]*	50	58%	36	44%	23%	33%	3%	64%	32%	27%	14%	4.0%
Klow N-E (1998)[22]	295	92%	n/r	no change in mean SCr			5%	59%	31%	40%	8%	0.7%
Total = 1179		84%	177	35%	53%	12%	12% (11%)	58% (56%)	30% (33%)	22%	13%	1.7%

*all patients with ostial renal artery disease, percentages in parenthresis are "intent to treat" values. PTRA = percutaneous transluminal renal artery angioplasty, n/r = not reported, SCr = serumcreatinine, HTN = hypertension.

unchanged and 12% worsened. Furthermore, restenosis was observed in 22% at variable follow-up.

In an effort to improve upon the outcome of PTRA, endoluminal stenting of the renal artery was developed. Although, currently no stent has been approved for renal use in the United States, the most common indications for their use appear to be: 1) elastic recoil of the vessel immediately after angioplasty, 2) renal artery dissection after angioplasty, and 3) restenosis after angioplasty. Recently, primary stenting of atherosclerotic renal artery disease has been reported. Review of published reports of percutaneous renal artery stenting reveals no improvement beyond PTRA alone with 61% of atherosclerotic patients experiencing blood pressure benefit while 25% experienced improvement in renal function (Table 2).[23–42] Restenosis was observed in 17% of patients at variable follow-up. When renal artery stenting was applied to ostial atherosclerotic renal artery stenosis in patients with ischemic nephropathy, only 17% experienced improvement in excretory renal function while restenosis was observed in 21% of patients (Table 3).[23,27–30,35,37,38,40,41] Consequently, for the majority of patients with ostial atherosclerosis in combination with renal insufficiency, we believe operative repair remains the best treatment. Nevertheless, the decision for interventional therapy for renovascular hypertension must be individualized. Patients who demonstrate significant and independent predictors of accelerated follow-up death (i.e., systolic dysfunction with clinical congestive heart failure, long-standing diabetes mellitus, uncorrectable azotemia) are considered for PTRA with or without stenting even when the renal artery lesions are suboptimal.

Operative Management

General Issues

The presence of hypertension is prerequisite for renal artery intervention. In general, functional studies are used to guide the management of unilateral lesions. Empiric renal artery repair is performed without functional studies when hypertension is severe, renal artery disease is bilateral or associated with ischemic nephropathy.[1] Accordingly, prophylactic renal artery repair in the absence of hypertension, whether as an isolated procedure or combined with aortic reconstruction, is not recommended. During surgical reconstruction, all hemodynamically significant renal artery disease is corrected in a single operation with the exception of bilateral ex vivo reconstructions which are staged. Having observed beneficial blood pressure and renal function response regardless of kidney size or histologic pattern on renal biopsy, nephrectomy is reserved for unreconstructable renal artery disease to a nonfunctioning kidney (i.e., $\leq$ 10% function by renography).[2] Direct aortorenal reconstructions are preferred over indirect methods since concomitant disease of the celiac axis is present in 40%–50% of patients and bilateral repair is required in half.[1] Because failed renal artery repair is associated with significantly increased risk of dialysis-dependence, intraoperative duplex is utilized to evaluate the technical results of surgical repair.[2,43]

Table 2.

Results after PTRA with Stent Placement for Atherosclerotic Renal Artery Stenosis.

Reference	Stent Type	Patients (n)	Technical Success (%)	Patients with Renal Dysfunction	Function Response after Angioplasty (%)			HTN Response after Angioplasty (%)			Reste-nosis (%)	Major Compli-cations (%)
					Improved	Unchanged	Worsened	Cured	Improved	Failed		
Rees CR (1991)[23]	Palmaz	28	96%	14	36%	36%	23%	11%	54%	36%	39%	18%
Wilms GE (1991)[24]	Wallstent	10	80%	1	0%	100%	0%	30%	40%	30%	22%	18%
Kuhn FP (1991)[25]	Strecker	8	92%	n/r	n/r	n/r	n/r	22%	34%	44%	17%	13%
Joffre F (1992)[26]	Wallstent	11	91%	4	50%	50%	0%	27%	64%	9%	18%	13%
Hennequin LM (1994)[27]	Wallstent	15	100%	6	20%	40%	40%	7%	93%	0%	27%	19%
Raynaud AC (1994)[28]	Wallstent	15	100%	7	0%	43%	57%	7%	43%	50%	13%	13%
MacLeod M (1995)[29]	Palmaz	28	100%	16	25%	75%		0%	40%	60%	17%	19%
van de Ven PJG (1995)[30]	Palmaz	24	100%	n/r	33%	58%	3%	0%	73%	27%	13%	13%
Dorros G (1995)[31]	Palmaz	76	100%	29	28%	28%	45%	6%	46%	48%	25%	11%
Henry M (1996)[32]	Palmaz	55	100%	10	20%	80%		18%	57%	24%	9%	3%
Iannone LA (1996)[33]	Palmaz	63	99%	29	36%	46%	13%	4%	35%	61%	14%	32%
Harden PN (1997)[34]	Palmaz	32	100%	32	35%	35%	29%	n/r	n/r	n/r	13%	19%
Blum U (1997)[35]	Palmaz	68	100%	20	0%	100%	0%	16%	62%	22%	17%	0%
Boisclair C (1997)[36]	Palmaz	33	100%	17	41%	35%	24%	6%	61%	33%	0%	21%
Rundback JH (1998)[37]	Palmaz	45	94%	45	18%	53%	33%	n/r	n/r	n/r	26%	9%
Fiala LA (1998)[38]	Palmaz	21	95%	9	0%	100%	0%		53%	47%	65%	19%
Dorros G (1998)[39]	Palmaz	163	99%	63	n/r	n/r	n/r	1%	42%	57%	n/r	14%
Tuttle KR (1998)[40]	Palmaz	120	98%	74	16%	75%	9%	2%	46%	52%	14%	4%
Gross CM (1998)[41]	*	30	100%	12	55%	27%	18%	0%	69%	31%	13%	n/r
Henry M (1999)[42]	#	200	99%	48	29%	67%	2%	19%	61%	20%	11%	2%
Total =		1045	98%	436	25%	57%	18%	9%	52%	39%	17%	10%

*Palmaz, Inflow, Sito and be-Stent; #Palmaz and Renal Bridge stents. PTRA = percutaneous transluminal renal artery angioplasty, n/r = not reported, HTN = hypertension.

Table 3.

Results after PTRA with Stent Placement for Ostial Atherosclerotic Renal Artery Stenosis.

Reference	Patients with Ostial Lesions (#)	Patients with Renal Dysfunction	Function Response after Angioplasty (%)			HTN Response after Angioplasty (%)			Restenosis (%)
			Improved	Unchanged	Worsened	Cured	Improved	Failed	
Rees CR (1991)[23]	28	14	36%	36%	29%	11%	54%	36%	39%
Hennequin LM (1994)[27]	7	2	0%	50%	50%	0%	100%	0%	43%
Raynaud AC (1994)[28]	4	3	0%	33%	67%	0%	50%	50%	33%
MacLeod M (1995)[29]	22	13	15%	85%		0%	31%	69%	20%
van de Ven PJG (1995)[30]	24	n/r.	33%	58%	8%	0%	73%	27%	13%
Blum U (1997)[35]	68	20	0%	100%	0%	16%	62%	22%	17%
Rundback JH (1998)[37]	32	32	16%	53%	31%	n/r	n/r	n/r	26%
Fiala LA (1998)[38]	21	9	0%	100%	0%	53%		47%	65%
Tuttle KR (1998)[40]	129	74	16%	75%	9%	2%	46%	52%	14%
Gross CM (1998)[41]	30	12	55%	27%	18%	0%	69%	31%	12%
Total =	365	179	17%	68%	15%	5%	55%	40%	21%

PTRA = percutaneous renal artery angioplasty, n/r = not reported, HTN = hypertension.

Preoperative Preparation

Antihypertensive medications are reduced during the preoperative period to the minimum necessary for blood pressure control. Patients requiring large doses of multiple medications will often have reduced requirements while hospitalized at bed rest. If continued therapy is required, vasodilators and selective β-adrenergic blocking agents are the agents of choice. If an adult's diastolic blood pressure exceeds 120 mmHg, operative treatment is postponed until the pressure is brought under control. In this instance, the combination of intravenous nitroprusside and esmolol is administered in an intensive care setting.

Operative Techniques

A variety of operative techniques have been used to correct renal artery disease. From a practical standpoint, three basic operations have been most frequently utilized: aortorenal bypass, renal artery thromboendarterectomy, and renal artery reimplantation (Table 4). Although each method may have its proponents, no single approach provides optimal repair for all types of renal artery disease. Aortorenal bypass, preferably with saphenous vein, is probably the most versatile technique, however, thromboendarterectomy is especially useful for ostial atherosclerosis involving multiple renal arteries. When the artery is sufficiently redundant, reimplantation is probably the simplest technique and one particularly appropriate to renal artery disease in children.

Certain measures are used in almost all renal artery operations. Mannitol is administered intravenously in 12.5 g doses early and repeated before and after periods of renal ischemia up to a total dose of 1 g/kg patient body weight. Just prior to renal artery cross-clamping, 100 units of heparin per kilogram body weight is given intravenously and systemic anticoagulation is verified by activated clotting time. Unless required for hemostasis, protamine is not routinely administered for reversal of heparin at the completion of the operation.

Table 4.

**Summary of Operative Management
1/87 Through 6/97
(n = 534 patients).**

Total renal reconstructions	720
Aortorenal bypass	445
Vein	288
PTFE	127
Dacron	19
Hypogastric artery	11
Ex Vivo	33
Reimplantation	52
Thromboendarterectomy	223
Total nephrectomies	57
Total kidneys operated	777

PTFE = polytetrafluoroethylene.

Provided the best method of reconstruction is selected for renal artery repair, the short course and high blood flow rates characteristic of renal reconstruction favor their patency. Consequently, flawless repair plays a dominant role in determining postoperative success. The impact of technical errors unrecognized and uncorrected at operation is implied by the fact that we have observed no late thromboses of renovascular reconstruction free of disease after 1 year.

The risks and the inherent limitations of completion angiography are not demonstrated by intraoperative duplex sonography. By placing the ultrasound probe immediately adjacent to the vascular repair, B-scan detail sensitive to < 1 mm anatomic defects is obtained. Once imaged, defects can be viewed in a variety of projections during conditions of uninterrupted, pulsatile blood flow. Intimal flaps not apparent during static conditions are easily imaged while avoiding the adverse effects of additional renal ischemia and potentially nephrotoxic contrast materials. In addition, important hemodynamic information is obtained from the spectral analysis of the Doppler-shifted signal proximal and distal to the anatomic defect. For these reasons, duplex sonography is the authors' preferred intraoperative method for assessing both renovascular and mesenteric repairs.

Results of Operative Repair

Demographics and Perioperative Management

From January 1987 through June 1997, 534 patients had operative renal artery repair at our center. Four hundred and fifty-four patients underwent repair for atherosclerotic renovascular disease while 80 patients were treated for nonatherosclerotic renovascular disease including congenital lesions and FMD. Unilateral procedures were performed in 269 patients and bilateral procedures in 265 for a total of 720 renal artery reconstructions.

Among atherosclerotic patients, there were 223 women and 231 men with a mean age of 65 ± 9 years. Their mean blood pressure was 197 ± 35/104 ± 22 mmHg with a mean duration of hypertension of 15 years. As a group, patients with atherosclerosis had widespread disease with 81% demonstrating at least one manifestation of cardiac disease including either angina, prior myocardial infarction, left ventricular hypertrophy, left heart strain on electrocardiogram or a prior coronary artery intervention. Thirty-four percent demonstrated a prior history significant for transient ischemic attack, cerebrovascular infarct or carotid endarterectomy. Finally, as evidenced by an SCr of 1.3 mg/dL or greater, 78% were considered to have at least mild renal insufficiency, including 37 patients dialysis-dependent. In all, 95% demonstrated at least one manifestation of subsystem damage. Among the 80 nonatherosclerotic patients, 58 were women and 22 were men. Their mean age was 58 ± 22 years with a mean duration of hypertension of 7 years (mean blood pressure: 194 ± 36/107 ± 20 mmHg).

Angiographic evaluation was performed in 95% of cases by cut-film angiography. These studies demonstrated bilateral renal artery disease in one-third of nonatherosclerotic patients and two-thirds of atherosclerotic patients.

Among atherosclerotic patients, renal artery disease was considered ostial in 97% of kidneys while 16% demonstrated renal artery occlusions.

Among 720 renal artery reconstructions, aortorenal bypass was performed in 445 instances with 288 vein grafts, 127 PTFE, 19 Dacron, and 11 hypogastric arteries (Table 4). Ex vivo repair was required in 35 instances while splanchnorenal bypass was performed in 6 instances. Renal artery reimplantation was performed in 52 instances while renal artery thromboendarterectomy was performed in 223 instances. There were a total of 57 nephrectomies for a total of 777 kidneys which underwent operation. Among atherosclerotic patients, 177 (40%) required simultaneous repair of clinically significant aortic disease.

Operative Morbidity and Mortality

Perioperative mortality as defined by in-hospital deaths or death within 30 days of surgery occurred in 18 patients (3.6%) (Table 5). All deaths occurred in older patients (mean age 67, range 64–70 years) with advanced atherosclerosis and were evenly divided among women and men. The cause of death was attributed to multiple organ failure in 10 patients, myocardial infarction/arrhythmia in 3, pneumonia in 2, cerebrovascular events in 2 and hemorrhage in 1. In addition, morbid events prolonging hospitalization occurred in 21% of these patients.

Blood Pressure Response

Using previously published criteria,[2] blood pressure and medication requirements at least 1 month after operative intervention were used to define blood pressure response. Among all surgical survivors, 89% were *cured* or *improved* while 11% were considered failed (Table 5). Although the proportion

Table 5.	
Results of Operation for Occlusive Renovascular Disease Among Surgical Survivors (n = 515 patients).	
	Percent
Perioperative Mortality	03.6
Hypertension Response	
Cured	18
Improved	71
Failed	11
Function Response*	
Improved	50
No Change	39
Worsened	11

*For 220 patients with preoperative serum creatinine ≥ 1.8 mg/dL; significant change ≥ 20% change in estimated glomerular filtration rate.

cured as compared with *improved* was higher among nonatherosclerotic patients, equivalent blood pressure benefit was observed for both atherosclerotic and dysplastic renal artery disease, irrespective of patient age, duration of hypertension, or extent of atherosclerosis.

Renal Function Response

A significant change in excretory renal function was defined as a change in estimated glomerular filtration rate (EGFR) of $\geq 20\%$ obtained at least 3 weeks after repair. Patients were classified as *improved* if they were removed from dialysis or if their EGFR increased by $\geq 20\%$. Patients were considered *worsened* if their EGFR decreased by $\geq 20\%$. All others were considered *unchanged*. Fifty percent of patients with a preoperative SCr ≥ 1.8 mg/dl were *improved* including 30 patients removed from dialysis (Table 5). Thirty-nine percent remained *unchanged* while 11% *worsened*. The proportion of patients *improved* increased with increasing severity of preoperative renal dysfunction with 81% of dialysis-dependent patients removed from dialysis. Subset analysis of patients with serial measurements of preoperative renal function suggested that the more rapid the rate of decline in renal function before surgery, the better

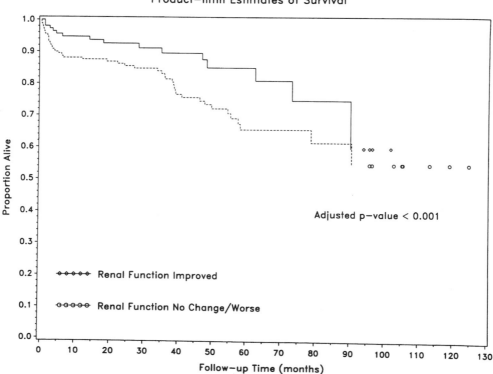

Figure 1. Product-limit estimates of overall survival after operative renal artery repair among atherosclerotic patients with improved excretory renal function compared with patients whose function remained unchanged or worsened.

the chance for recovery of function after operation. Improved renal function was significantly associated with the site of disease and the extent of repair. One-third of patients demonstrated improved renal function after unilateral repair, however, when considered as groups, only bilateral repair was associated with a significant increase in EGFR.

Significance of Blood Pressure and Renal Function Benefit

At a mean follow-up of 34 months, an additional 71 patients died, all in the atherosclerotic group. By product-limit estimate, beneficial blood pressure response was not associated with improved estimated survival compared with patients considered failed (p = 0.956). In contrast, renal function response to operative repair influenced both survival and eventual dialysis-dependence. Compared with patients unchanged or worsened, patients with improved renal function demonstrated a significant and independent association with improved survival (p < 0.001, Figure 1). Improved renal function in response to operation was significantly and independently associated with improved dialysis-free survival (p < 0.001, Figure 2) as well as decreased risk for dialysis-dependence (p < 0.001, Figure 3). Patients whose renal function remained un-

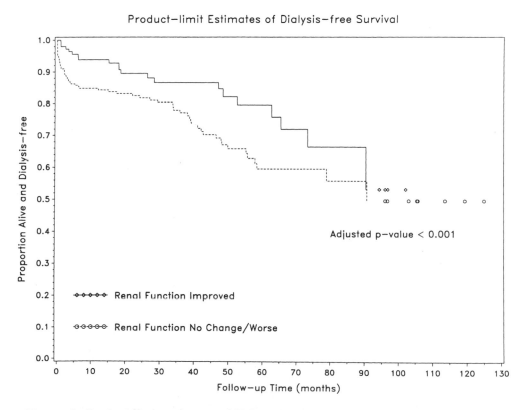

Figure 2. Product-limit estimates of dialysis-free survival after operative renal artery repair among atherosclerotic patients with improved excretory renal function compared with patients whose function remained unchanged or worsened.

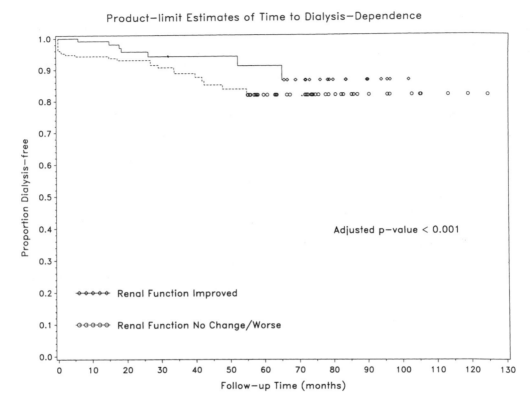

Product−limit Estimates of Time to Dialysis−Dependence

Figure 3. Product-limit estimates of time to dialysis-dependence after operative renal artery repair among atherosclerotic patients with improved excretory renal function compared with patients whose function remained unchanged or worsened.

changed demonstrated a relative risk of follow-up dialysis-dependence and death that approached that of patients worsened after surgery.

Operative Failures and Consequences of Secondary Repair

Among all 534 patients, at mean follow-up of 27 months, a failed renal artery repair was identified in 20 patients, 12 with recurrent hypertension and 8 with recurrent hypertension and worsening excretory renal function.[2] This subgroup included 9 women and 11 men, ranging in age from 12 to 77 years (mean: 54 years) treated for either FMD (6 patients), atherosclerotic renovascular disease (13 patients) or coarctation of the abdominal aorta. Prior to primary renal artery reconstruction, each patient had hypertension (mean blood pressure: 198/111 mmHg; mean medications: 3 drugs) and preoperative SCr ranged from 0.7 to 3.3 mg/dL (mean: 1.6 mg/dL). Evidenced by an SCr $\geq$ 1.8 mg/dL off high dose diuretics and converting enzyme inhibitors, 7 patients were considered to have renal dysfunction, including 1 patient dependent on dialysis. Failed PTRA preceded primary operative intervention in 4 patients (1 FMD; 3 with atherosclerotic renovascular disease).

Blood pressure response after secondary operative intervention was equivalent to that observed among 514 patients with primary operative intervention only (Table 6). Among 17 patients after primary operative intervention, 4 (24%) patients were classified as *cured*, 12 (70%) patients were classified as *improved*, and 1 (6%) patient was classified as *failed*. Considering all 20 patients after secondary operation, 3 (15%) patients were classified as *cured*, 16 (80%) patients were classified as *improved*, and 1 (5%) patient was classified as *failed*. Beneficial blood pressure response (i.e., *cured* and *improved*) demonstrated no association with type of renal artery disease and was equivalent for patients receiving nephrectomy or secondary renal artery reconstruction.

Renal function response after primary renal artery repair demonstrated 10 (59%) patients *improved*, including 1 patient removed from dialysis-dependence, 5 (29%) patients were *unchanged*, and 2 (12%) patients were classified as *worsened*. Secondary renal function response differed significantly from the function response observed among 514 patients treated with primary repair only (p = 0.015, Table 6). Eventual renal function response in all 20 patients after secondary operative intervention was classified as *improved* in 2 (10%) patients, *unchanged* in 10 (50%) patients, and *worsened* in 8 (40%) patients, including 7 patients dependent upon dialysis. Considering only patients with atherosclerotic renovascular disease, 1 patient was *improved*, 5 were *unchanged*, and 7 were eventually dialysis-dependent. Eventual renal function response was not associated with the extent of primary renal artery disease or renal artery repair, renal artery thrombosis or stenosis, or secondary renal artery repair or nephrectomy. However, eventual renal function response demonstrated a significant association with the presence of ischemic nephropathy (i.e., SCr ≥1.8 mg/dL) prior to the first procedure (p= 0.039) and bilateral failure of primary repair (p = 0.007).

Table 6.

Comparison of Eventual Results of Secondary Intervention (n = 20) with Results From Primary Intervention Only (n = 514).

	Primary Intervention Only	Secondary Intervention		P Value
		Initial	Eventual	
Perioperative Mortality (%)	3.6%	0%	0%	NS
Hpertension Response (%)				
Cured	19%	24%	15%	NS
Improved	71%	70%	80%	
No Change	10%	6%	5%	
Renal Function Response (%)				
Improved	34%	59%	10%	0.003
No Change	53%	29%	50%	
Worsened	13%	12%	40%	
Eventual Dialysis-Dependence	4%	0%	35%	< 0.001

NS = no significant difference.

Patients requiring secondary renal artery intervention had a significantly greater risk of worsened renal function (40% vs. 13%; p = 0.015), including eventual dialysis-dependence (35% vs. 4%; p < 0.001). Furthermore, patients requiring secondary intervention demonstrated a significant risk for decreased dialysis-free survival (RR: 2.4; C.I.: 1.1, 5.4; p = 0.035).

This experience with failed renal artery repairs reinforces two important issues. First, significant hypertension is considered a prerequisite to renovascular intervention.[44] The irretrievable loss of excretory renal function observed after failed renal artery repair supports the view that renal revascularization should be performed for clear clinical indications, not as a "prophylactic" procedure in the absence of either hypertension or renal insufficiency. Second, the direct aortorenal reconstructions utilized in these patients are characterized by their short length and high blood flow, favoring prolonged patency. Early failures of repair reflect errors in surgical technique or judgment. To recognize and eliminate these technical errors, intraoperative renal duplex sonography has been performed as a completion study in the last 266 consecutive patients (unpublished data). Overall, 12% of 377 renal artery repairs demonstrated major technical defects which were immediately revised. As a result, early failure of repair has occurred in only 2 (0.5%) of these last 377 renal reconstructions.

The use of PTRA after failed renal artery intervention deserves comment. In this series, PTRA was utilized in 7 of 20 patients prior to either primary (4 patients; 6 arteries) or secondary (3 patients; 5 arteries) operative intervention. In the case of failed operative repair, the technical challenges posed by secondary operative intervention, may make PTRA appealing. Although widely applied to a variety of renal artery lesions, little information is available regarding the immediate or long-term results of PTRA after failed operative intervention.[45–47] In this group, PTRA was applied to 5 renal arteries after primary operative repair stenosed by a sclerotic venous valve, focal subendothelial fibrous proliferation, or recurrent disease at a site of endarterectomy. In each case, PTRA was considered immediately successful but failed 1 to 8 months later. In one instance, a secondary stenosis progressed to thrombosis after PTRA and required nephrectomy. Given the paucity of data regarding PTRA after failed operative repair, secondary operative intervention should be considered the preferred, albeit challenging, method of remedial management.

Surgery after Failed Percutaneous Transluminal Renal Artery Angioplasty

With these results in mind, we recently reviewed our experience with 32 consecutive atherosclerotic patients repaired after a prior failed PTRA (F-PTRA).[48] We examined the influence of failure of PTRA on methods of secondary surgical management, and blood pressure and excretory renal function response to operation.

From January 1987 through June 1998, 571 consecutive patients underwent operation for renovascular disease at our center. Of the 473 patients treated for atherosclerotic renovascular disease, 32 had surgical repair after F-

PTRA in 36 renal arteries. Twenty-five patients had unilateral and 7 had bilateral PTRA (including 2 solitary kidneys). Four patients had repeat PTRA and three patients had renal artery stents placed. These patients included 19 females and 13 males (mean age: 61.2 ± 9.5 years; range: 33 to 78 years). Prior to PTRA, 31 patients had significant hypertension (mean blood pressure: 188 ± 32/102 ± 15 mmHg) and 19 patients had ischemic nephropathy (mean SCr: 2.0 ± 1.3 mg/dL; range: 1.3 to 6.6 mg/dL). After F-PTRA, 3 of 32 patients required emergent intervention for acute renal artery thrombosis, renal artery rupture or renal artery stent infection with septic pseudoaneurysm. The remaining 29 patients had elective operation for either recurrent (28 patients), or persistent (1 patient) hypertension (mean preoperative blood pressure: 205 ± 34/110 ± 23 mmHg; mean medications: 2.5 ± 1.1). Twenty patients had ischemic nephropathy after F-PTRA (mean SCr: 2.0 ± 0.8 mg/dL; range: 1.3 to 4.1 mg/dL [excluding 2 patients dialysis-dependent]). Excluding the 3 emergency operative procedures, the interval between F-PTRA and surgical repair ranged from 3 weeks to 12 years (mean: 24.8 ± 32.6 months; median: 9 months).

Forty-three atherosclerotic kidneys were surgically repaired, 32 had repair after F-PTRA and 11 contralateral renal arteries were repaired simultaneously. Including 3 emergency operations, secondary operative repair was considered complicated by F-PTRA in 19 patients (59% of atherosclerotic patients). In 6 patients periarterial fibrosis after F-PTRA resulted in a technically more difficult dissection and prolonged repair. More distal branch renal artery exposure and reconstruction was required in 10 patients (3 with associated periarterial fibrosis) and nephrectomy of a previously reconstructable kidney was required in 3 patients. In all, 4 nephrectomies were required after F-PTRA. Bilateral procedures were performed in 20 patients including repair of 2 solitary kidneys and unilateral procedures were performed in 12 patients. Aortorenal bypass was performed in 25 instances (21 saphenous vein, 4 PTFE), splenorenal bypass in 2 and an ex vivo bypass in 1 instance. Renal artery reimplantation was performed in 6 instances. Ten renal artery thromboendarterectomies were performed by either transrenal (9 instances) or transaortic (1 instance) techniques. Combined aortic reconstruction was performed in 3 patients (1 AAA, 1 occlusive disease, 1 infection).

On mean follow-up of 42 ± 38 months, 9 additional deaths occurred. Two of these patients had progressed to dialysis-dependent end-stage renal disease. A third patient remains alive on dialysis. In all, 3 atherosclerotic patients progressed to dialysis-dependence. These 3 patients represent 3 of 4 patients (75%) who required nephrectomy after F-PTRA. Late graft thrombosis (3%) occurred in 1 patient at 15 months. Although the proportion of atherosclerotic patients treated for F-PTRA progressing to death or dialysis-dependence was significantly greater than the patients treated by operative repair alone (40.6 vs. 20.5%; p = 0.013), this difference reflected different mean follow-up (42.3 ± 37.8 vs. 28.3 ± 27 months). By product-limit estimate, there was no difference in follow-up death or dialysis-dependence (p = 0.668). However, when considering only atherosclerotic patients requiring nephrectomy, there was a significantly greater incidence of dialysis-dependence after F-PTRA compared with operative repair alone (p < 0.001).

Blood Pressure Response

Among 28 operative survivors with atherosclerotic renovascular disease and hypertension repaired after F-PTRA, 2 patients (7%) were considered *cured*, 14 patients (50%) *improved*, and 12 patients (43%) were *failed* (Table 7). Compared with patients treated by operative repair only, F-PTRA was associated with significantly decreased blood pressure benefit (57% vs. 89% benefited; p < 0.001).

Renal Function Response

Among 17 operative survivors with preoperative renal insufficiency, 7 patients (41%) were considered *improved* including 1 patient removed from dialysis-dependence. Ten patients (59%) were *unchanged*. Compared with patients treated with operative repair only, the proportion of patients with *improved* renal function after surgery were similar (p = 0.804; Table 7).

When considering all 28 operative survivors with atherosclerotic renovascular disease repaired after F-PTRA, preoperative EGFR compared with postoperative EGFR was significantly increased (47.4 ± 4.2 vs. 56.6 ± 5.1 mL/min/1.73m^2; p = 0.002). Applying model-based estimates of EGFR to allow for multiple statistical comparisons, the decline in EGFR before balloon dilatation compared to preoperative EGFR after F-PTRA (51.6 ± 3.4 vs. 47.4 ± 3.9 mL/min/1.73m2) was not statistically significant (p = 0.152; Table 8). Over-

Table 7.

Comparison of Operative Intervention after F-PTRA versus Primary Operative Intervention Alone for Atherosclerotic Renovascular Disease.

	Primary Operative Intervention Only (%)	Secondary Operative Intervention after F-PTRA (%)	P Value
Perioperative mortality	4.3	9.4	NS
Hypertension response			
Cured	11	7	< .001
Improved	78	50	
No change	11	43	
Renal function response			
(Preop SCr > 1.3 mg/dL)			
Improved	47	41	NS
No change	43	59	
Worsened	10	0	
Eventual dialysis-			
dependence	7.2	9.4	NS
Follow-up death rate	18.4	37.5	.018*

*differences not significant by life-table analysis.

F-PTRA = failed percutaneous transluminal renal artery angioplasty; Preop SCr = preoperative serum creatinine;

NS = no significant difference.

Table 8.

Comparison of EGFR for Atherosclerotic Patients with F-PTRA.

Procedure: PTRA/Operative Repair	n	PrePTRA EGFR ± SE	Preoperative EGFR ± SE	P Value#	Postoperative EGFR ± SE	P Value**
Overall	28	51.6 ± 3.4*	47.4 ± 3.9	0.152	56.6 ± 4.9	0.121
Unilateral/Unilateral	11	48.4 ± 5.3	51.4 ± 6.2	0.486	63.3 ± 7.8	0.005
Unilateral/Bilateral	12	50.7 ± 5.1	44.1 ± 6.0	0.122	45.7 ± 7.5	0.282
Bilateral/Unilateral	1	68.7 ± 17.7	94.5 ± 20.7	–	94.5 ± 26	–
Bilateral/Bilateral	4	58.6 ± 10.2*	34.6 ± 10.3	0.232	61.1 ± 13	0.79

*modeled EGFR.
#prePTRA EGFR vs. preoperative EGFR.
**prePTRA EGFR vs. postoperative EGFR.
##Note: P = 0.012 for Overall: preoperative EGFR vs. postoperative EGFR.
EGFR = estimated glomerular filtration rate in mL/min/1.73 m²; F-PTRA = failed percutaneous transluminal renal artery angioplasty; Unilateral = unilateral procedure; Bilateral = bilateral procedure; SE = standard error of the mean.

all, the change in EGFR from before balloon dilatation compared to postoperative EGFR was not different (51.6 ± 3.4 vs. 56.6 ± 4.9 mL/min/1.73m2; p = 0.121).

In contrast with previous reports by McCann[49] and Martinez[50], our experience with operative management after F-PTRA was characterized by periarterial fibrosis and increased complexity of repair. Eighty-percent of balloon dilatations described in this experience were considered an immediate technical success, with recurrence months after the initial percutaneous treatment. In the case of atherosclerosis, initial success of PTRA is often associated with focal dissection of the renal artery lesion and disruption of the internal elastic lamina.[51] Similar to spontaneous renal artery dissection, these events are frequently associated with early perivascular inflammation and eventual periarterial fibrosis. Alternatively, percutaneous treatment after an inability to cross a renal artery lesion and elastic recoil may not be associated with this perivascular response. Regardless of the presence of these perivascular changes, we consider the requirement for more distal branch renal artery repair after F-PTRA and emergent renovascular procedures for rupture or thrombosis as increased in complexity.

This experience demonstrated decreased blood pressure benefit among atherosclerotic patients after operative repair for F-PTRA when compared with primary surgical intervention alone, however, the explanation for this difference is uncertain. The observed result may reflect the limitations of surgical repair, PTRA, or both. Failed balloon angioplasty was associated with branch renal artery exposure and more distal, branch renal artery reconstruction. Although failure of secondary surgical repair was detected infrequently (3%), branch disease contributing to hypertension may have been underestimated. Conversely, the eventual blood pressure response after secondary operative repair may reflect limitations of PTRA. Although considered an immediate technical success in 80% of instances, hemodynamic assessment of percutaneous treatment was performed infrequently. Angiographic appearance may correlate poorly with residual pressure gradient or evaluation by intravascular ultrasound. In addition, percutaneous dilatation may be associated with distal atheroembolization. By creating occlusion and activation of the renin-angiotensin axis at the microvascular level, renal artery repair may fail to provide blood pressure benefit.

Assessment of initial renal function response after PTRA was impossible, as renal function data was not routinely obtained after percutaneous dilatation. Nevertheless, when compared with EGFR prior to secondary operative repair, initial renal function declined after F-PTRA. Although surgical repair led to a significant increase in excretory renal function, compared with renal function prior to PTRA, there was no change. Whether patients treated after F-PTRA should be considered improved or unchanged with regard to renal function is not certain. However, this distinction may have importance when the change in EGFR after intervention is compared with the subsequent decline in excretory function and the progression to dialysis-dependence. Considering all atherosclerotic patients treated at our center since January of 1987, only those patients with a significant (i.e., $\geq 20\%$) increase in EGFR after surgical renal artery repair demonstrated a significant decrease in the rate of decline in renal function, as well as, a significant and independent increase in dialysis-free survival.[2] Patients whose renal function remained unchanged demonstrated a relative risk of follow-up dialysis-dependence and death equivalent to patients worsened after surgery.[8] The common practice of reporting unchanged renal function as "preserved" after renovascular intervention is misleading. Patients with ischemic nephropathy unchanged after intervention remain at increased risk for eventual dialysis-dependence and death.[1,8]

Conclusions

With proper patient selection and preparation, operative repair of atherosclerotic renovascular disease results in both blood pressure and renal function benefit. Improvement in renal function is associated with a significant increase in dialysis-free survival independent of other co-morbidities. The application of intraoperative duplex to assess renal artery reconstruction has resulted in long-term patency exceeding 96%. However, when failure of operative repair does occur, eventual renal function is worsened culminating in increased risk of dialysis-dependence and death.

Percutaneous transluminal angioplasty with and without stenting offers similar blood pressure benefit for medial fibroplasia of the main renal artery and nonostial atherosclerotic lesions. However, for suboptimal lesions, especially in the presence of ischemic nephropathy, PTRA with or without endoluminal stenting yields inferior renal function benefit. In addition, the requirements of repair after a failed angioplasty are not insignificant. Our experience demonstrates increased complexity of repair as well as an inferior blood pressure benefit. Whether renal function can be considered *improved* relative to initial function remains unclear. For these reasons, the authors recommend operative repair of ostial atherosclerosis and renal artery occlusion associated with severe hypertension and renal insufficiency.

References

1. Hansen KJ, Starr SM, Sands RE, et al. Contemporary surgical management of renovascular disease. *J Vasc Surg* 1992; 16:319–331.
2. Hansen KJ, Deitch JA, Oskin TC, et al. Renal artery repair: Consequence of operative failures. *Ann Surg* 1998; 227:678–690.
3. Lawson JD, Boerth RF, Foster JH, et al. Diagnosis and management of renovascular hypertension in children. *Arch Surg* 1977; 112:1307–1316.
4. Svetkey LP, Bollinger RR, Kotman PE, et al. Prospective analysis of strategies for diagnosing renovascular hypertension. *Hypertension* 1989; 14:242–257.
5. Nally JV Jr, Chen CC, Skakianakis G, et al. Diagnostic criteria of renovascular hypertension with captopril renography: A consensus statement. *Am J Hypertens* 1991; 4:749S-752S.
6. Dean RH, Benjamin ME, Hansen KJ: Surgical management of renovascular hypertension. *Curr Probl Surg* 1997; 34(3): 209–308.
7. Hansen KJ, Tribble RW, Reavis S, et al. Renal duplex sonography: Evaluation of clinical utility. *J Vasc Surg* 1990; 12:227–236.
8. Dean RH, Tribble RW, Hansen KJ, et al. Evolution of renal insufficiency in ischemic nephropathy. *Ann Surg* 1991; 213:446–455.
9. Hansen KJ, Thomason RB, Craven TE, et al. Surgical management of dialysis-dependent ischemic nephropathy. *J Vasc Surg* 1995; 21:197–209.
10. Hansen KJ, Benjamin ME, Appel RG, et al. Renovascular hypertension in the elderly: Results of surgical management. *Geriatr Nephrol Urol* 1996; 6:3–34.
11. Hunt JC, Strong CG: Renovascular hypertension. Mechanisms, natural history and treatment. *Am J Cardiol* 1973; 32:562–574.
12. Dean RH, Kieffer RW, Smith BM, et al. Renovascular hypertension: Anatomic and renal function changes during drug therapy. *Arch Surg* 1981; 166:1408–1415.
13. Canzanello JC, Millan VG, Spiegel JE, et al. Percutaneous transluminal renal angioplasty in management of atherosclerotic renovascular hypertension: Results in 100 patients. *Hypertension* 1989; 13:163–172.
14. Klinge J, Mali WP, Puijlaert CB, et al. Percutaneous transluminal renal angioplasty: Initial and long-term results. *Radiology* 1989; 171:501–506.
15. Baert AL, Wilms G, Amery A, et al. Percutaneous transluminal renal angioplasty: Initial results and long-term follow-up in 202 patients. *Cardiovasc Intervet Rad* 1990; 13:22–28.
16. Tykarski A, Edwards R, Dominiczak AF, et al. Percutaneous transluminal renal angioplasty in the management of hypertension and renal failure in patients with renal artery stenosis. *J Hum Hypert* 1993; 7:491–496.
17. Weibull H, Bergqvist D, Bergentz SE, et al. Percutaneous transluminal renal angioplasty versus surgical reconstruction of renal artery stenosis: A prospective randomized study. *J Vasc Surg* 1993; 18:841–850.
18. Losinno F, Zuccala A, Busato F, et al. Renal artery angioplasty for renovascular hypertension and preservation of renal function: Long-term angiographic and clinical follow-up. *Amer J Rad* 1994; 162:853–857.
19. Rodriguez-Perez JC, Plaza C, Reyes R, et al. Treatment of renovascular hypertension with percutaneous transluminal angioplasty: Experience in Spain. *J Vasc Interv Rad* 1994; 5:101–109.
20. Bonelli FS, McKusick MA, Textor SC, et al. Renal artery angioplasty: Technical results and clinical outcomes in 320 patients. *Mayo Clin Proc* 1995; 70:1041–1052.
21. Hoffman O, Carreres T, Sapoval MR, et al. Ostial renal artery stenosis: Immediate and mid-term angiographic and clinical results. *J Vasc Interv Rad* 1998; 9:65–73.
22. Klow N-E, Paulsen D, Vatne K, et al. Percutaneous transluminal renal artery angioplasty using the coaxial technique: Ten years of experience from 591 procedures in 419 patients. *Acta Rad* 1998; 39:594–603.
23. Rees CR, Palmaz JC, Becker GJ, et al. Palmaz stent in atherosclerotic stenosis involving the ostia of the renal arteries: Preliminary report of a multicenter study. *Interv Rad* 1991; 181:507–514.

24. Wilms GE, Peene PT, Baert AL, et al. Renal artery stent placement with use of the Wallstent endoprosthesis. *Radiology* 1991; 179:457–462.
25. Kuhn FP, Kutkuhn B, Torsello G, et al. Renal artery stenosis: Preliminary results of treatment with the Strecker stent. *Radiology* 1991; 180:367–372.
26. Joffre F, Rousseau H, Bernadet P, et al. Midterm results of renal artery stenting. *Cardiovasc Interv Radiology* 1992; 15:313–318.
27. Hennequin LM, Joffre FG, Rousseau HP, et al. Renal artery stent placement: Long term results with the Wallstent endoprosthesis. *Radiology* 1994; 191:713–719.
28. Raynaud AC, Beyssen BM, Turmel-Rodrigues LE, et al. Renal artery stent placement: Immediate and midterm technical and clinical results. *J Vasc Interv Rad* 1994; 5:849–858.
29. MacLoed M, Taylor AD, Baxter G, et al. Renal artery stenosis managed by Palmaz stent insertion: Technical and clinical outcome. *J Hypert* 1995; 13:1791–1795.
30. Van de Ven PJG, Beutler JJ, Kaatee R, et al. Transluminal vascular stent for ostial atherosclerotic renal artery stenosis. *Lancet* 1995; 346:672–674.
31. Dorros G, Jaff M, Jain A, et al. Follow-up of primary Palmaz–Schatz stent placement for atherosclerotic renal artery stenosis. *Am J Card* 1995; 75:1051–1055.
32. Henry M, Amor M, Henry I, et al. Stent placement in the renal artery: Three-year experience with the Palmaz stent. *J Vasc Interv Rad* 1996; 7:343–350.
33. Iannone LA, Underwood PL, Nath A, et al. Effect of primary balloon expandable renal artery stents on long-term patency, renal function, and blood pressure in hypertensive and renal insufficient patients with renal artery stenosis. *Cathet Cardiovasc Diagn* 1996; 37:243–250.
34. Harden PN, MacLoed MJ, Rodger RSC, et al. Effect of renal artery stenting on progression of renovascular renal failure. *Lancet* 1997; 249:1133–1136.
35. Blum U, Krumme B, Flugel P, et al. Treatment of ostial renal artery stenosis with vascular endoprostheses after unsuccessful balloon angioplasty. *New Eng J Med* 1997; 336:459–465.
36. Boisclar C, Therasse E, Oliva VL, et al. Treatment of renal artery angioplasty failure by percutaneous renal artery stenting with Palmaz stents: Midterm technical and clinical results. *Amer J Rad* 1997; 168:245–251.
37. Rundback JH, Gray RJ, Rozenblit G, et al. Renal artery stent placement for the management of ischemic nephropathy. *J Vasc Interv Rad* 1998; 9:413–420.
38. Fiala LA, Jackson MR, Gillespie DL, et al. Primary stenting of atherosclerotic renal artery ostial stenosis. *Ann Vasc Surg* 1998; 12:128–133.
39. Dorros G, Jaff M, Mathiak L, et al. Four-year follow-up of Palmaz-Schatz stent revascularization as treatment for atherosclerotic renal artery stenosis. *Circulation* 1998; 98:642–647.
40. Tuttle KR, Chouinard RF, Webber JT, et al. Treatment of atherosclerotic ostial renal artery stenosis with the intravascular stent. *Am J Kidney Dis* 1998; 32(4): 611–622.
41. Gross CM, Kramer J, Waigand J, et al. Ostial renal artery stent placement for atherosclerotic renal artery stenosis in patients with coronary artery disease. *Cathet Cardiovasc Diagn* 1998; 45:1–8.
42. Henry M, Amor M, Henry I, et al. Stents in the treatment of renal artery stenosis: Long-term follow-up. *J Endovasc Surg* 1999; 6:42–51.
43. Hansen KJ, O'Neil EA, Reavis SW, et al. Intraoperative duplex sonography during renal artery reconstruction. *J Vasc Surg* 1991; 14:364–374.
44. Benjamin ME, Hansen KJ, Craven TE, et al. Combined aortic and renal artery surgery: A contemporary experience. *Ann Surg* 1996; 233:555–565.
45. Libertino JA, Beckmann CF: Surgery and percutaneous angioplasty in the management of renovascular hypertension. *Urol Clin North Am* 1994; 21(2): 235–243.
46. Novick AC: Percutaneous transluminal angioplasty and surgery of the renal artery. *Eur J Vasc Surg* 1994; 8:1–9.
47. Erdoes LS, Berman SS, Hunter GC, et al. Comparative analysis of percutaneous transluminal angioplasty and operation for renal revascularization. *Am J Kidney Dis* 1996; 27(4): 496–503.

48. Wong JM, Hansen KJ, Oskin TC, et al. Surgery after failed percutaneous renal artery angioplasty. *J Vasc Surg* 1999; 30:468–483.
49. McCann RL, Bollinger RR, Newman GE. Surgical renal artery reconstruction after percutaneous transluminal angioplasty. *J Vasc Surg* 1988; 8:389–394.
50. Martinez AG, Novick AC, Hayes JM. Surgical treatment of renal artery stenosis after failed percutaneous transluminal angioplasty. *J Urol* 1990; 144:1094–1096.
51. Lyon RT, Zarins CK, Lu CT, et al. Vessel, plaque, and lumen morphology after transluminal balloon angioplasty-Quantitative study in distended human arteries. *Arteriosclerosis* 1987; 7:306–314.

5

The Techniques of Performing Endovascular Renal Artery Stenting

Kenneth Rosenfield, MD and Robert F. Fishman, MD

Introduction

Percutaneous revascularization of renal arteries has been performed for over two decades, and has now superceded surgical revascularization as the treatment of choice under all but a few circumstances. The situations where surgery is the preferred modality are now limited to the occasional patient with renal artery occlusion that cannot be traversed, an aorta that is known to have excessively friable plaque, or an anatomically inaccessible renal artery. Absent these findings, revascularization via percutaneous transluminal renal angioplasty (PTRA) can be expected to achieve technical success in greater than 95% of cases.[1-7] However, in spite of this high degree of technical success, clinical success is less reliably achieved.[8,9] Much of the reason for this discrepancy between angiographic success and clinical/physiologic success is not yet understood. It is likely due to the multi-factorial etiology of nephropathy and hypertension; because of this ambiguity, it is nearly impossible to predict in advance of revascularization to what degree the nephropathy or hypertension is due to renal artery stenosis versus other nonremediable factors, and what the clinical outcome will be. Nonetheless, what has become apparent is that procedural success is not dependent upon simply getting the artery open. Perhaps more than most other percutaneous procedures, the care, precision, and attention to detail exercised during the intervention greatly influences the outcome. The simple explanation for this is that the target organ is often already diseased

From Jaff MR (ed): *Endovascular Therapy for Atherosclerotic Renal Artery Stenosis: Present and Future*. Armonk, NY: Future Publishing Co, Inc.; ©2001.

and very vulnerable to additional insults. Since the kidney arises from the abdominal aorta in a site which is notoriously laden with friable atherosclerotic plaque, atheroembolization of any amount can be detrimental, if not outright catastrophic, to the very organ one seeks to salvage.[10–12] Similarly, the contrast agents used to visualize the renal artery during revascularization can be harmful.

Achieving technical success in opening a renal artery, but trashing the kidney with cholesterol emboli or overwhelming it with contrast, is tantamount to "winning the battle but losing the war." In order to win the war, one must carefully select the appropriate candidates for revascularization, be knowledgeable of the anatomy and its variants, be well-versed in the technique and equipment used in PTRA and stenting, and perform the intervention cautiously. Anticipation of complications is perhaps the most important factor in avoiding them, and thereby optimizing outcome.

The state of the art of renal stenting, as with many endovascular procedures, is evolving rapidly. Since the pioneering work of Gruntzig, who first reported the technique of renal balloon angioplasty in 1978,[13] and Tegtmeyer,[14] there has been an ongoing evolution in the technology of guidewires, balloons, guiding catheters, sheaths, and stents. Advantages in all of these technologies have improved the safety and efficacy of this procedure. While sharing many of

---

Table 1.

PTRA—Guiding Principles for Renal Intervention.

- Select patients carefully and appropriately
  - avoid "incidental" renal angiography during other studies (e.g. cardiac cath), unless appropriate indications present
  - know anatomy and physiology in the patient: blood pressures, overall renal function, size of kidneys, and relative function of each kidney.
- Perform nonselective angiography in advance of selective cannulation, to:
  - identify status of aorta
  - identify origins of all renal arteries
  - delineate nephrogram
  - facilitate selective renal artery cannulation with minimal manipulation
- Avoid trauma in abdominal aorta
  - minimize manipulation
  - select catheters carefully, based on configuration of aorta and location/orientation of renal arteries
  - have full range of catheters available in inventory
  - avoid direct cannulation with guiding catheter; transition it over less traumatic diagnostic catheter
- Minimize contrast
- Hydrate patient before and after procedure
- Measure pressure gradient before dilation, to confirm physiological significance of lesion (unless stenosis is critical)
- Avoid over-sizing balloons (use IVUS if question about vessel size)
- Monitor patient for pain during inflations; stop inflating when patient has pain
- "Protect" stent, to ensure successful delivery and avoid stent embolization
- Compare final nephrogram to baseline, to ensure no change

the same principles, the technique of renal artery stenting is distinctly different from that used in other vascular trees, such as the coronary circulation. The major difference is due to the anatomic relationship of the renal artery to the abdominal aorta which supplies it. The propensity for atherosclerotic plaque to deposit immediately adjacent to the renal artery makes local manipulation more hazardous than is the case in, for example, coronary angioplasty. This single fact underlies many of the principles that must be upheld for successful renal intervention (Table 1). This chapter will attempt to guide vascular interventionalists in the appropriate and safe techniques involved in renal artery angioplasty and stenting.

Lesion Site Definition

Percutaneous transluminal angioplasty of atherosclerotic renal artery stenosis (ARAS) has been less successful than in patients with fibromuscular dysplasia (FMD). The major reason for this reduced efficacy lies in the differences in the underlying pathology. Patients with medial FMD have dense fibrous ridges alternating with thin aneurysms of the vessel wall. The acute and long-term results with PTRA of these lesions after therapeutic disruption of the fibrous bands by balloon inflation has been favorable. In contrast, atherosclerotic lesions are bulkier, more commonly calcified, often aorto-ostial in location, and thus more resistant to balloon inflation. In addition, these lesions are more prone to immediate or delayed elastic recoil and unfavorable long-term remodeling after balloon angioplasty. Thus, the immediate success rates from initial series were suboptimal, and restenosis rates were high.[8,15] Over the past decade, however, numerous investigators have reported on the utility of stent placement for ARAS with very encouraging acute and long-term results.[5,16,17]

The distribution of atherosclerotic plaque within the renal artery may extend from the aorta to the distal branches. Most commonly, however, the plaque involves the aorto-ostium or the proximal portion of the renal artery. Plaque may also be found at bifurcation points within the renal vascular tree. Lesion location plays an important role in the outcome of percutaneous interventions. Cicuto and colleagues[18] noted that lesions located within the renal artery responded very well after PTRA, while lesions that involved the aorta did not. The authors suggested that bulky plaques at the renal artery orifice are more prone to recoil after PTRA, due to the orientation of the elastic and collagen fibers in the muscularis and adventitial layers of the aorta. Plaques along the aortic wall are simply displaced and not compressed by balloon inflation. Kaatee and colleagues further refined the definition of aorto-ostial lesions by comparing digital subtraction angiograms with spiral CT angiography.[19] The authors noted that some lesions that were thought to only involve the trunk of the renal artery actually began within the aorta. They noted that there was an infundibulum of the aorta at the level of the origin of the renal artery, suggesting that these lesions were truly aorto-ostial. These "pseudo-truncal" stenoses respond to PTRA more like aorto-ostial stenoses, with less favorable acute and long-term results than lesions within the body of the renal artery. The authors suggested that lesions that originate within 10 mm of the aorta be classified as ostial lesions. Appropriate classification of lesion location is therefore extremely important when comparing results of various trials.

Invasive Approaches and Techniques

Access

Renal artery stenting can be performed using either the retrograde brachial or femoral arterial approach. Each has advantages and disadvantages (Table 2). The choice of access site is influenced by the pathology and orientation of the renal arteries as assessed by the prior diagnostic angiogram or other imaging study (magnetic resonance angiography [MRA] or Duplex scan), presence of atherosclerotic disease, tortuosity, and abnormalities of the abdominal aorta and iliac vessels. The major advantage to the brachial approach is to minimize contact with the infrarenal abdominal aorta, which may be riddled with friable atherosclerotic plaque. In addition, the brachial approach is preferred for obtaining a coaxial catheter and stent position to facilitate stent delivery in arteries which are oriented cephalad (Figure1). There was more compelling reason to introduce stents coaxially, however, in the bygone era when only rigid

Table 2.

Access for Renal Stent Deployment.

	Advantages	Disadvantages	Required

Femoral	Familiarity
	Short distance to target
	Catheter exchange easier
	More pre-shaped guides
	  available
	Selective cannulation easier
	Avoidance of brachiocephalic
	  vessels (reduced chance of
	  stroke)
	Ability to easily treat other
	  disease (e.g., iliac)
	  simultaneously
		Possibility of disruption
		  of atheromatous plaque
		  in diseased infrarenal aorta
		Avoidance of AAA
		Difficult stent delivery in
		  severely angulated
		  renal artery origin	

Brachial	Potential avoidance of AAA
	  or friable plaque in
	  infra-renal aorta
	Obtain coaxial guide and
	  stent position in
	  down-going renal artery
		Small caliber brachial artery
		Smaller target for arteriotomy
		More vascular complications
			occluded
			infrarenal
			aorta

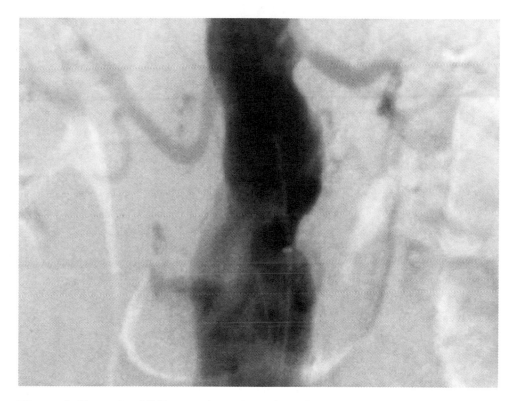

Figure 1. Example of different orientations of renal artery (RA). Left RA has stenosis, with horizontal orientation, easy to access from femoral approach. Right RA, however, has cephalad orientation, with acute "hair-pin" turn at origin. If this vessel required placement of stent- especially earlier rigid models—it could be problematic from femoral approach. Current generation of flexible, low-profile stents may be more deliverable.

stents were available. Current technology, with flexible stents which adhere well to their delivery systems, enable traversal of even the most acute bends at the renal artery origin. Thus, concerns about deliverability and dislodgment are now less pertinent. The major disadvantages of the brachial approach are the limitation in size of sheaths and catheters that can be used in the smaller brachial artery, the requirement for longer sheaths and catheters that are more difficult to manipulate, and a higher percentage of complications related to vascular access. Most interventionalists currently prefer the femoral approach, unless the abdominal aorta is occluded (Figure 2) or there is a particularly down-going takeoff of the renal artery. Also, in rare instances, an unusual configuration of plaque within a severe ostial lesion renders access from below impossible, in which cases the brachial approach is the only percutaneous alternative. Finally, some prefer brachial access if the infra-renal aorta is known to have friable plaque or an aneurysm harboring a large amount of thrombus. In such instances, it should be made clear that brachial access in and of itself is not protective against atheroembolism.

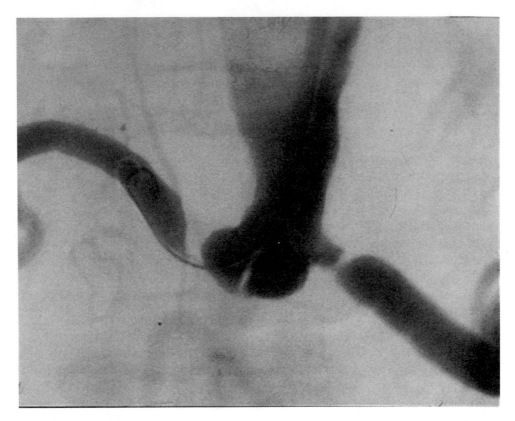

Figure 2. Example of patient with bilateral renal artery stenosis with co-existing occlusion of infrarenal aorta. Brachial (or radial) access is required for stenting of these vessels.

Cannulation of the Renal Artery

The original technique of PTRA, as described by Tegtmeyer and Sos[14,20] did not entail use of a guiding catheter. Following nonselective angiography of the abdominal aorta and renal arteries, selective cannulation of the renal artery was performed using a diagnostic catheter. A guidewire was then passed across the lesion and the diagnostic catheter was then exchanged for the balloon angioplasty catheter. The lesion was dilated, and then the balloon was removed. The guidewire was also often removed, and angiography was again performed nonselectively from the abdominal aorta, to ascertain the result of the intervention. The disadvantage of this technique is that diagnostic angiography cannot be performed during positioning of the balloon catheter and the stent. Instead, bony landmarks are used to identify the correct position. Furthermore, guidewire position must be sacrificed in order to ascertain the outcome of the intervention. If angiography is necessary or desired for balloon (or stent) localization, or if one wishes to maintain guidewire position, a second catheter may be placed in the abdominal aorta via the contralateral femoral artery.[3] However, this requires additional access. Finally, another disadvantage of this technique is that passage of the balloon catheter and/or stent may be difficult, due to the lack of backup support. In spite of these limitations, some interventionalists continue to prefer this approach.

Gruntzig developed a guiding catheter system for PTRA; however, these were large catheters (9 Fr) bulky and stiff, and could easily damage the aortic wall during manipulations. White and colleagues[21] described the use of 8 Fr, soft-tipped angiographic guiding catheters to perform PTRA. These guiding catheters had an internal lumen diameter of 0.082" and were available in five shapes, including a multi-purpose curve, a short and long-tipped renal double curve, and a hockey stick. The guiding catheters simplified diagnostic angiography during the intervention, provided excellent backup for insertion of the balloon catheters and stents, facilitated the use of dual guidewires to protect side branches, and afforded the opportunity to measure simultaneous translesional pressure measurements to assess the hemodynamic effect of balloon dilatations, all through a single arterial access site.

Today, while some continue to use the technique described by Tegtmeyer and Sos, most high volume interventionalists prefer the guiding catheter technique to perform renal stenting. Because of the atherosclerotic nature of the aorta and the variable location of the renal artery origin, care must be exercised, and certain principles adhered to, during use of these stiff guiding catheters during renal intervention. Adherence to these principles will ensure optimal outcomes and fewer complications.

PTRA and Stenting from the Femoral Approach

The femoral approach is favored when the renal arteries are oriented horizontally or caudally with respect to the aorta. In many laboratories, it is the preferred approach in all cases, irrespective of orientation of the renal artery, as long as the infrarenal aorta is not occluded. Vascular access is typically obtained using a 6, 7, or 8 Fr sheath, advanced under direct fluoroscopic control over a 0.035 inch guidewire. Prior to performing renal artery intervention, it behooves the operator to become familiar with the features of the equipment required for the procedure, including the full range of choices available. It also is helpful to develop a strategy in advance, so as to minimize procedure time, contrast dose, and manipulation within the aorta.

Role of Nonselective Angiography

Nonselective angiography is highly recommended prior to selective cannulation of the renal artery and other branches which arise off the abdominal aorta. There are several important reasons for this recommendation (Table 3). First, nonselective angiography provides valuable information regarding the configuration of the aorta, the presence or absence of an abdominal aortic aneurysm and, the overall size and orientation of the aorta (which should influence the selection of both diagnostic and guiding catheters). Secondly, nonselective angiography delineates the location and orientation of the renal ostia. Armed with this knowledge, and also with the information regarding the size

---

Table 3.

Value of Nonselective Aorto-renal Angiography
Before Selective Cannulation.

- Obtain information about aortic configuration
  - size
  - shape
  - orientation
- Identify Renal Arteries
  - number of vessels
  - presence of accessory renal arteries
  - location and orientation
  - preliminary assessment of degree of stenosis (location of plaque, etiology of stenosis)
- Assess size of kidneys and configuration of nephrogram
- Identify important aortic pathology
  - AAA
  - Friable plaque
- Facilitate choice of selective diagnositic and guiding catheters
- Minimize complications

---

and configuration of the aorta, the appropriate diagnostic catheter can be chosen for selective angiography, and manipulation within the abdominal aorta can be minimized. Thirdly, nonselective angiography identifies the presence or absence of anatomic variants, such as dual renal supply or accessory renal arteries. Fourth, abdominal aortography may at times exclude the diagnosis of renal artery stenosis, thus obviating the need for selective cannulation.

One potentional disadvantage of nonselective abdominal aortography is the requirement for an additional contrast injection. In patients with severe renal insufficiency, in whom every drop of contrast may be deleterious, contrast dose can be minimized by diluting the injectate and by shortening the injection time. For example, a 60% contrast solution can be further diluted by 25% or 30%, and injected at 15 cc per second for a total of 15 or 20 cc. Therefore, the total contrast injected is minimized, and yet the information provided can be more than adequate. In these instances, if substraction angiography is used and the technique and set-up is appropriate, the essential information (origin of the renal arteries, general configuration of the aorta, presence or absence of accessory branches) can usually be obtained with this amount of contrast. The catheter must also be placed at the correct level, so as to minimize contrast "spillage" into the celiac and superior mesenteric arteries (SMAs) (see below).

A number of catheters, in 4, 5, or 6 Fr diameters are available for nonselective angiography (Figure 3). While a conventional pig-tail catheter can be used, this configuration often leads to retrograde flow of contrast, spilling over to the SMA or celiac artery. Since some of the main branches of the SMA tend to overlap and obscure the origins of the renal arteries, it is preferable not to fill these more cephalad visceral vessels. Specialized catheter configurations (e.g. tennis racket and omni-flush) offer the advantage of more lateral and less retrograde/cephalad contrast flow, which results in reduced filling of the SMA. In order to optimize imaging, however, even these catheters must be placed at

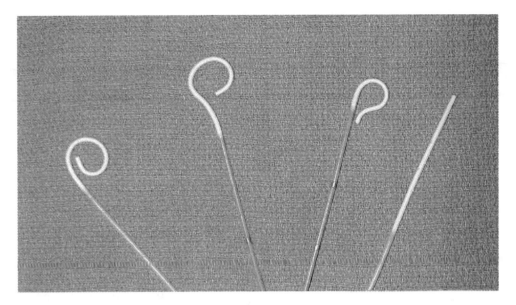

Figure 3. Catheters used for nonselective aorto-renal angiography. Left to right: conventional pigtail, tennis racquet, omni flush, straight flush with multiple side holes. Tennis racquet and omni flush catheters disperse contrast laterally and therefore offer advantage of less retrograde/cephalad contrast flow. Thus, opacification of the celiac and superior mesenteric arteries can be minimized.

the appropriate level, usually lining up the top of the catheter with the top of the first lumbar vertebral body (Figure 4). Also, the appropriate contrast dosage and injection rate must be used. Typically, 20 to 30 cc of dye is injected at a rate of between 10 and 17 cc per second, which is generally sufficient to demonstrate the origins of the renal arteries and the configuration of the aorta without completely opacifying the SMA and celiac. A larger aorta may require more volume and/or higher injection rate. Likewise, a hypoplastic aorta might require less. In a patient with severe renal insufficiency, as mentioned above, one can identify the renal ostia with as little as 10 to 15 cc of dilute contrast material. Some interventionalists utilize CO_2 or Gadalinium in order to minimize contrast exposure.

Selective Angiography

Selective angiography is required to best define the degree of disease in the renal artery. Whether for diagnostic purposes alone, or as the first step in an intervention, direct cannulation of the renal artery should be carried out as atraumatically as possible. Accordingly, it is recommended that the initial selective angiography be performed using a soft-tipped, 4, 5, or 6 Fr diagnostic catheter (as opposed to a guiding catheter). Various shapes are available, and should be selected based on the size and configuration of the aorta and the orientation of the renal artery(s) (Figure 5). Some commonly used catheter curves include an internal mammary, Judkins right 4, renal double curve (RDC), Sos

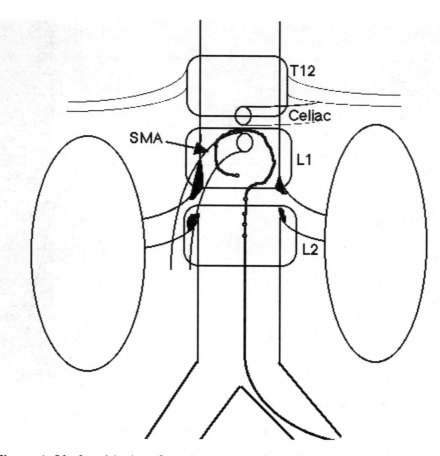

Figure 4. Ideal positioning of tennis racquet catheter for nonselective imaging of renal arteries. Positioning the top of the catheter at or near the top of the first lumbar vertebral body usually results in excellent visualization of renal arteries, without opacifying the superior mesenteric artery (SMA). If filled, the SMA may obscure pathology at the origin of either renal artery.

omni, hockey stick, multi-purpose, and cobra. Each of these curves also can be ordered with different tip lengths and subtle variations. The soft smaller diagnostic catheter is used first, rather than the guiding catheter, so as to minimize trauma to the aorta, which could precipitate cholesterol embolization. Caution must be exercised, however, even in manipulation of the least traumatic catheters, as they too can liberate atheroemboli.

If intervention is planned, to save time, the diagnostic catheter can be "pre-loaded" by advancing it through a rotating hemostatic y-adapter attached to a 6, 7, or 8 Fr renal guiding catheter (size chosen to match the anticipated stent to be deployed). (Figure 6). The guiding catheter is kept in the distal abdominal aorta, away from the renal ostium, during manipulation of the softer diagnostic catheter and performance of diagnostic angiography.

Diagnostic angiography should not only include the appropriate views of the renal artery and the lesion, but also should include a careful assessment of

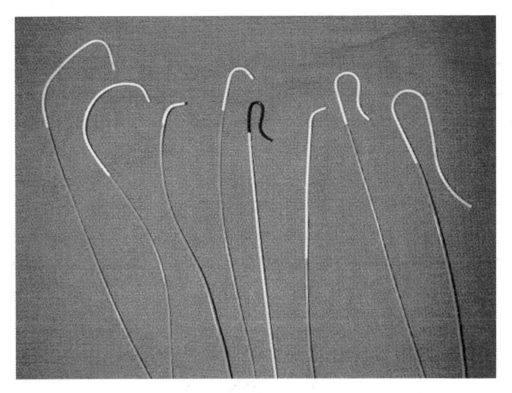

Figure 5. Diagnostic catheter shapes commonly used for selective cannulation and angiography of renal arteries. Left to Right: renal double curve, cobra, Judkins right, left internal mammary, Sos omni, Berenstein, Simmons1, Simmons2.

the baseline nephrogram. Thus, alterations in the nephrogram post-procedure may elucidate peri-renal (e.g., subcapsular hematomas, perforations, or fistula) formation, which might have developed during the intervention.

To perform PTRA, a guidewire is then carefully inserted into the renal artery through the diagnostic catheter. Ideal 0.035 inch wires, which are atraumatic, soft-tipped, and steerable, yet provide adequate support, include the Wholey wire (Mallinkrodt, St. Louis, Missouri), the Storque wire (Cordis Corporation, Miami, Florida) and the Magic Torque wire (Boston Scientific Corporation, Watertown, Massachusetts). If the vessel is critically narrowed or there is significant irregularity of the plaque at the ostium, precluding the passage of a 0.035 inch wire, a 0.014 inch or 0.018 inch guidewire system can be used. In general, hydrophilic guidewires should be avoided during renal intervention, due to the risk of dissection and distal perforation.

Once the lesion has been traversed, the diagnostic catheter is advanced across the lesion. If the lesion is noncritical, the diagnostic catheter usually passes easily across the lesion. For more critical or calcific lesions, a 4 Fr or hydrophilic catheter may be required. On occasion, the diagnostic catheter will not cross the lesion, and predilation with a lower profile 0.014" or 0.018"-based coronary or small-vessel peripheral balloon is required. The method of advancement of the diagnostic catheter varies, depending on the type of catheter

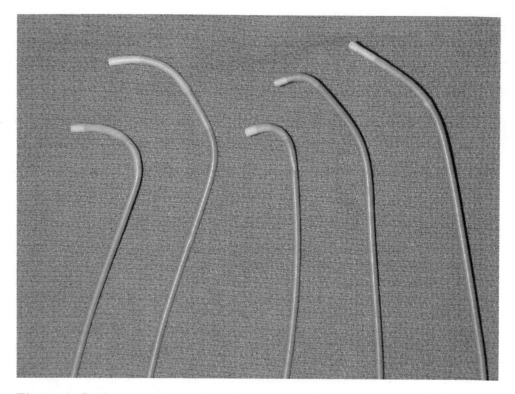

Figure 6. Guiding catheter configurations commonly used in renal angioplasty and stenting. Left to Right: Hockey Stick (HS), Renal double curve (RDC), Left Internal Mammary (LIMA), Renal double curve 1 (RDC1), Multipurpose.

used. For the internal mammary, Judkins right 4 and Cobra catheters, one pushes the catheter forward, while holding the guidewire position constant. However, if a Sos Omni or Simmons catheter is used, due to the retroflexed shape of these catheters, pulling back on the catheter while fixing the guidewire in place will advance the catheter across the lesion.

Pressure Gradient Measurement

Once the diagnostic catheter is across the lesion, the guidewire can be removed and a pressure gradient established across the lesion (measured between the diagnostic catheter beyond the lesion, and the guiding catheter in the distal aorta). Pressure gradients can be measured before angioplasty and after stenting to determine the efficacy of the procedure.[22,23] The gradient is typically measured using a 4 or 5Fr angiographic catheter. Measurement via the distal aspect of the balloon catheter is less reliable, due to the additional space occupied by the balloon itself. The gradient is measured (preferably simultaneously) distal to the lesion and in the aorta, close to the renal ostium. A significant gradient is, by convention, considered to be a pressure differential greater than 10 mmHG mean or 20 mmHG peak. Provocation of a significant gradient can be obtained by injecting nitroglycerin (200 or 300 micrograms), or another vasodilator, downstream via the distal catheter; although the true significance of a provoked gradient is unknown. Likewise, the conventional wisdom regarding what constitutes a "significant" resting gradient is not based on any solid data. Dorros has hypothesized that complete abolishment of the trans-stenotic pressure gradient is likely to be clinically important.[18] In renovascular hypertension, renin is continuously released in response to renal artery pressure. Therefore, as Dorros suggested, the failure of PTRA to reduce blood pressure may be due to the inability of angioplasty alone to abolish the pressure gradient. He showed that stenting was more effective at abolishing the pressure gradient than angioplasty alone. Ongoing studies will hopefully verify this hypothesis.

The *absence* of any baseline resting gradient is considered to be strong evidence that revascularization will have little beneficial effect either on blood pressure or acute renal function. So, the absence of a baseline pressure gradient should signal the end of a procedure, unless there is compelling evidence otherwise that revascularization is indicated. Such an instance might be the presence of a 70% stenosis in a vessel supplying a solitary kidney, with recent progression in the degree of stenosis. Absent such a scenario, it is the opinion of the authors that intervention should be avoided if no pressure gradient is detectable when measured through a 4 or 5 Fr diagnostic catheter. There is no data yet available analyzing gradients obtained using "pressure-sensing guidewires" which have recently become available.

Guide Catheter Positioning

Following pressure measurements, an appropriate guidewire is reintroduced and the guiding catheter is carefully advanced to the level of the renal ostium over the diagnostic catheter, using the latter to transition the guide into place. Utilizing this coaxial technique, the guiding catheter itself is not manipulated within the abdominal aorta. The diagnostic catheter is then removed, leaving the guidewire in place and the guiding catheter situated close to the renal ostium. Care must be taken at this point, however, to maintain the guiding catheter in a coaxial position with respect to the guidewire and the renal artery. Unlike the performance of guiding catheters used for coronary interventions, there is virtually 1:1 responsiveness of renal artery guides. The reason for this difference is primarily the fact that a coronary guiding catheter traverses the aortic arch and has contact with the aorta in multiple sites. The friction provided by these contact sites minimizes the effect on the catheter tip of a small rotation applied at the level of the groin. In contrast, the renal artery guiding catheter has no such contacts with the aorta as it travels en route to the renal artery. This, plus the short length of the catheters, leads to a situation where minimal twisting or rotation of the catheter outside the body will be directly conveyed to the tip of the catheter. While this sensitivity can be a benefit in terms of responsiveness, it can also be a liability. The combination of guide catheter responsiveness and absence of availability of good guidewire anchoring position in the renal artery bed can lead to a sudden disengagement and loss of guidewire position. Thus, the interventionalist should be careful at all times to maintain stable and coaxial guide catheter position.

Balloon Dilation

Dilation with a balloon angioplasty catheter is then performed. When stenting is planned, predilation is usually carried out, in order to facilitate stent delivery and reduce the likelihood of the stent being stripped off of the balloon delivery system. To minimize the possibility of causing a large dissection, a slightly under-sized balloon can be used. This has the secondary benefit of confirming the renal artery diameter before committing to a given stent size and length. Another advantage to predilation is to ensure that the vessel is "dilatable." There are rare instances in which the calcific nature of the lesion precludes adequate dilation. In those instances, surgical revascularization may be required. In undilatable lesions, we have had success on occasion using rotation atherectomy to facilitate subsequent balloon angioplasty. Some interventionalists prefer to deliver the stent without predilation. This can be done in cases of moderate disease; but in critical lesions, there is a significant chance of encountering difficulty with traversal of lesion, or achieving precise stent localization, as well as a greater likelihood of "stent stripping" and embolization. Nonetheless, the current generation of premounted stents, which are tightly bound or adherent to their balloons, does lend itself well to "direct stenting." The appropriate choice of balloon catheter size can be made using quantitative angiography or intravascular ultrasound (IVUS). As mentioned, the predilation balloon can assist in estimating renal artery size. If these measurements are not available, then balloon size can be estimated by comparing the diameter of the guiding catheter to that of the reference segment beyond the stenosis in the renal artery. In general, the main renal artery is between 6 and 8 mm for a man, and between 5 and 7 mm for a woman. However, many patients fall outside of those "norms", especially if the kidney is supplied by more than one vessel. The balloon is inflated so as to eliminate the waste caused by the lesion. Care should be taken not to overdilate the renal artery, otherwise rupture can ensue. *During each inflation, the patient should be specifically asked if he/she is experiencing discomfort.* If the patient complains of more than mild flank or abdominal pain during inflation, this suggests that the balloon may be oversized, or certainly at the upper limit. The discomfort should decrease immediately following balloon deflation; continued intense pain following deflation suggests the presence of renal artery rupture. If, on initiation of inflation, the patient develops intense pain that decreases rapidly with balloon deflation, it may be wise to exchange for a smaller balloon catheter before inflating to higher pressure.

Following predilation the guiding catheter is atraumatically advanced over the balloon as it is deflated. This maneuver positions the guide beyond the lesion, thus protecting the stent during its subsequent delivery. The movement required for this technique is simply to advance the guiding catheter during balloon deflation, while fixing the balloon catheter in place. Utilizing the newer, low profile 0.018" and 0.014" systems, with premounted stents, this maneuver may not be as crucial. However, in the case of hand-mounted stents advanced over a 0.035" guidewire, the guiding catheter advancement beyond the lesion is an essential maneuver to avoid stent dislodgement and embolization during delivery.

Orientation of X-ray Tube and C-Arm

Prior to deploying the stent, efforts should be made to optimize the imaging of the aorto-ostial junction. It is preferable to view the origin of the renal artery *"en face."* In a normal, pre-atherosclerotic aorta, the renal arteries arise from the postero-lateral aspect of the aorta. Thus, optimal *"en face"* imaging of the left renal artery would be in the LAO projection, and the right renal artery would be in the RAO projection. However, this typical orientation may be completely altered due to tortuosity, elongation, ectasia, and other distortions within the diseased abdominal aorta. Administration of small test doses of contrast in multiple projections via the nonselective catheter may help to determine the optimal angle for a formal diagnostic angiogram. However, concern about contrast overdosing often limits the number of injections possible at this and later stages. Accordingly, it is adequate for the nonselective study to identify the level (e.g., "latitude") of the origin of the renal arteries, even if the circumferential angle ("longitude") is suboptimal and the vessels are not visualized well enough to characterize or assess the degree of disease. Armed with the appropriate "latitudinal" information, selective cannulation can then be carried out with minimal manipulation and scraping (e.g., "windshield wiping") within the aorta. Another method for identifying the correct orientation is to adjust the C-arm while the balloon is in place, either inflated or deflated. When adjusting the C-arm, if one searches for the angle in which the balloon (located within the lesion) is most elongated, then that orientation is usually ideal for viewing the lesion and the aorto-ostial junction. Thus, without administration of any contrast, one can identify the orientation of takeoff of the renal artery and, likely, the optimal view for stent deployment.

Stent Selection

Following removal of the predilatation balloon, an appropriately sized stent is then mounted on an angioplasty balloon catheter. In the current era, many of these stents are premounted and, therefore, the appropriate length and diameter must be selected. The stent should be crimped extremely tightly on the balloon, taking care not to damage either the stent or the balloon. When using a premounted stent, the stent should be inspected carefully to ensure that there has not been any damage.

As stated earlier, the technology and equipment available for renal angioplasty and stenting has evolved rapidly, even within the past year. During this time, novel stents have become available that are both flexible and low profile, yet offer radial strength (hoop strength) that is superior to their more rigid predecessors. Some of these devices are now available on a 0.014" or 0.018" premounted platform. This enables the use of 7 and 6 Fr guiding catheters, which are much less treacherous and traumatic to the aorta. In addition, these low profile premounted stents often can be passed across stenoses without predilatation (as mentioned) and enable the use of 0.018" or 0.014" guidewires – often required to cross tight stenoses at the beginning of a case anyway – to be utilized for the full duration of the procedure. For specific stents that are currently used during renal stenting, please refer to Table 4. Most interventionalists prefer balloon-expandable stents for this application, due to the increased precision with which they can be placed over their self-expanding cousins. The authors believe that self-expanding stents have not, as of this time, been proven to be as effective as balloon-expandable stents in the renal artery. It is further worth noting that, in the United States as of January 2001, no stent has yet received United States Food and Drug Administration (FDA) approval for use in renal arteries. The stents described in Table 4 are all approved for biliary applications and therefore available commercially in the United States. Several FDA-approved trials are currently underway to gain approval for stenting in renal applications. It is anticipated that approval will be obtained at some time within the near future.

Stent Deployment

The stent delivery system is advanced through a widely open hemostatic valve, while holding the stent firmly, until it has entered the guiding catheter. The stent is then advanced and positioned across the lesion and the guiding catheter is subsequently withdrawn into the aorta, exposing the stent. The balloon/stent assembly has a tendency to be "sucked" into the renal artery as the guide is withdrawn; simultaneous application of gentle negative force on the balloon catheter prevents this from occurring. Careful angiography is performed to ensure appropriate positioning of the stent, taking into account the

---

Table 4.

**Stents Used for Renal Artery
Revascularization (2001)**

Cordis (Miami, FL)
    Palmaz "04 series" (104,154,204,294,394)
    Palmaz long medium (424,564,784)
    Corinthian IQ
Intratherapeutics (ITI) (St. Paul, MN)
    Single strut
    Double strut
Medtronics/AVE (Santa Rosa, CA)
    Bridge Stent
Guidant (Santa Clara, CA)
    Megalink
    Herculink
Boston Scientific/Medinol (Watertown, MA)
    NIR Peripheral

---

anticipated shortening of the stent when expanded. In addition, for ostial lesions, the stent needs ultimately to extend beyond the ostium into the aorta approximately 0.5–2.0 mm after deployment. It should be noted that vigorous angiography with certain stent-balloon combinations may force the stent off the balloon. The stent is then deployed generally peaking at 9–12 atmospheres of pressure. Gradual inflation should be used, so as to create a "dumbbell" or "dog bone" appearance to the balloon. This will prevent stent migration, which can otherwise occur during asymmetric balloon inflation. For ostial lesions, the balloon is withdrawn and the ostium is postdilated to higher pressures. A larger balloon may be necessary to flare the stent at the ostium. Care should be taken not to overdilate the distal nonstented vessel. Dissections beyond the stent can easily propagate into the distal branches. Likewise, discomfort in the flank or abdomen during inflation should serve as a warning not to push to higher pressure or larger balloons.

The stent delivery balloon is then withdrawn into the guiding catheter. It is critical not to disrupt the stent with the guiding catheter when the stent is placed in the ostium of the renal artery. If the guiding catheter has migrated inferiorly into the aorta, withdrawing the stent delivery balloon will pull the catheter towards the RA ostium and potentially cause the guiding catheter to crush the stent. The guiding catheter can be kept coaxial to the stent and away from the protruding struts at its inferior edge by either: 1) inflating the balloon to low pressure within the stent and gently advancing the guide over the balloon catheter (e.g., "transitioning" the guide over the deflating balloon); 2) turning the guiding catheter posteriorly and then advancing the guide while turning it towards the renal ostium; or 3) "over-advancing" a soft-tipped guidewire into the distal vessel to disengage (e.g., "kick out") the guide, and then readvance the guide over the "extended" wire. The last technique pushes the guide off the aortic wall, but at the expense of deep-seating a guidewire in the distal renal bed. The technique can be very effective, but must be performed cautiously and certainly must not be used if a hydrophilic guidewire is in place.

Further balloon dilation may be required based on angiographic results, IVUS, or pressure gradient measurements. Prior to insertion of balloon catheters through the stent, care must be taken to ensure the guiding catheter is coaxial. Final angiography is then performed with careful attention to the distal vasculature and nephrogram making certain that neither has been altered. The guiding catheter is then removed over the guidewire.

Brachial Approach

Due to the smaller caliber of the brachial artery, guiding catheters are generally not used from this approach. A 5.5 to 7.5 Fr, 70–90 cm long vascular sheath is introduced in conjunction with a 4 to 6 Fr multipurpose or Judkins right diagnostic catheter over a 0.035" guidewire into the abdominal aorta. Baseline angiography is performed as above. The procedure is similar to that performed via the femoral approach, however, the access sheath acts as the guiding catheter. After predilation, the sheath is advanced across the lesion over the balloon catheter. The stent delivery system is then advanced through the sheath to the lesion and the sheath is withdrawn into the aorta. Angiography is performed via the sheath, instead of a guiding catheter.

Intravascular Ultrasound

IVUS can be useful before and after percutaneous procedures in the renal vasculature.[24] IVUS determination of reference vessel size is helpful in sizing balloons and stents. This is particularly true for the coronary interventionalist who may not be accustomed to gauging arterial sizes in the periphery. IVUS provides useful data on lesion characteristics such as calcification, lesion length, and involvement and exact location of the ostium. Postprocedurally, IVUS is helpful in revealing stent underexpansion, stent asymmetry, and distal vessel dissection, all of which may be angiographically occult. In addition, if guidewire position is lost after stent deployment, IVUS can ensure proper positioning of the guidewire after reintroduction. For patients with severe renal insufficiency, IVUS-guided percutaneous intervention may also enable significant reduction in total dye load, which clearly benefits this patient population.

Definition of Success

A problem that plagues the literature in percutaneous renal procedures is the lack of consistency in the definition of success. A successful PTRA (without stenting) has variably been defined as residual stenosis < 50% or < 30%, with a peak-to-peak pressure gradient < 20 mmHg without major complications. There is no generally agreed upon definition of success after stenting. It has been suggested that a successful stent procedure requires < 30% residual stenosis by angiography and complete elimination of the trans-stenotic pressure gradient, without major complications.

Periprocedure Care

Patients should receive vigorous hydration before, during, and after the procedure. Pretreatment with aspirin is necessary prior to stent placement. Some operators add a thiopyridine such as clopridogrel or ticlopidine to their pre- and poststent regimen. No data is currently available regarding their use in the renal circulation. Most operators use nonionic contrast during PTRA and stenting. Heparin is administered after sheath insertion, prior to angioplasty. Typically, a bolus of 70 units/kg is administered to achieve an activated clotting time of approximately 250 seconds during the procedure. No further heparin is administered post-procedure and oral anticoagulation with warfarin is not required. The arterial sheaths are removed when the activated clotting time is less than 170 seconds. Glycoprotein 2B3A inhibitors are not routinely used in most laboratories during PTRA/stenting.

There is a considerable range of opinion regarding management of antihypertensive medications given periprocedurally. Some interventionalists withhold all blood pressure medications, and then add them back one at a time postprocedure. Others prefer not to change therapy until after successful revascularization, at which time the medicines are withdrawn one at a time, based upon blood pressure readings and renal function. There is no universal agreement as to the optimal approach, but there is agreement that careful monitoring of the patient's blood pressure postprocedure is mandatory. Consideration of the individual patient's anatomy and clinical status may shed light on the response to revascularization. For example, patients with "global renal ischemia" (i.e. bilateral renal artery stenosis or unilateral stenosis in a solitary kidney) who undergo PTRA may exhibit a precipitous decline in their blood pressure. In such situations, consideration should be given to reducing anti-hypertensive medications pre-procedure and careful adjustment is required postprocedure. In general, long-acting medications should be changed to shorter acting preparations on the day of the procedure. Careful follow-up of the creatinine and electrolytes is required.

Complex Lesion Subsets

Ostial Lesions

As discussed earlier in this chapter, aorto-ostial lesions tend to have a greater plaque burden, are more resistent to balloon inflation, are prone to plaque shift as opposed to plaque compression, and respond less well to balloon inflation alone. Stenting appears to be the procedure of choice for aorto-ostial lesions as the stent can scaffold the artery, reduce elastic recoil, plaque shift, and prevent unfavorable remodeling and thus reduce restenosis. Stent placement must be precise in the renal ostium. If the stent is deployed slightly too distally, there would be no beneficial effect on the ostium. If the stent is placed with excessive metal outside the renal ostium, subsequent attempts at engaging the renal ostium may be quite difficult.

The operator must therefore be certain of the location of the renal ostium. Conventional anteroposterior angiograms may not adequately delineate the renal ostium. The operator may be fooled by the angiogram and position the stent inappropriately. Individualized oblique views, possibly in conjuction with IVUS may best define the renal ostium.

Bifurcation Lesions

It is not uncommon for the renal artery to bifurcate in its proximal third, or even at its origin, a site typical for atherosclerosis. Both angioplasty and stenting techniques have been described for renal bifurcation lesions. The difficulty in bifurcation angioplasty is that of the "snow-plow" effect. When the balloon is inflated in one branch, the plaque shifts into the nondilated branch. Typically, simultaneous balloon inflation ("kissing balloon angioplasty") is required to reduce the likelihood of plaque shifting. Simultaneous inflation is feasible through using an 8-Fr guiding catheter, using a combination of 0.014"/0.018"-based coronary and peripheral angioplasty balloons. If larger balloons are required, dual access, either femoral and brachial, or bilateral femoral, may be necessary.[25] Bifurcation stenting can entail "T-stenting," "Y-stenting," or "culotte stenting." In general, stent designs with open interstices are favored when performing bifurcation stenting, thus allowing for passage of guidewires, balloons, and stents through the struts for side-branch dilation.[26]

Bilateral Renal Artery Stenosis

It has been suggested that simultaneous revascularization of bilateral renal artery stenosis is associated with higher complications.[20] Sos has recommended revascularization of the larger and technically easier kidney, then adopting a wait-and-see approach for the other kidney. Clearly, if one kidney measures < 8cm, revascularization is not likely indicated. As mentioned, if both kidneys are revascularized at the same time or a solitary kidney is revascularized, careful attention must be paid to the contrast dose, post-procedure blood pressure and renal function. Revascularization in patients with "global renal ischemia" may occasionally cause a precipitous drop in blood pressure, although this usually responds to vigorous hydration.

Total Occlusions

Percutaneous revascularization of total occlusions can be performed,[27] albeit at higher risk. This risk is not only related to the ipsilateral kidney, but also extends to the contralateral kidney and the mesenteric vessels, which could be embolized while manipulating within the aorta to find the renal ostium. Also, it is not uncommon for a cleft in the aorta to be mistaken for the renal ostium, and for aortic plaque to be disrupted and/or stained by contrast injection. While these events are not necessarily associated with complications or poor outcomes, they certainly can be and should thus be avoided. Sos has recommended that angioplasty for total occlusion not be attempted in most patients who have normal renal function and an ipsilateral kidney size < 8–9cm. When considering recanalization of an occluded renal artery, given the excess risk, the merits of the alternative therapies (renal artery bypass or additional medical therapy) must be carefully evaluated. PTRA should be reserved for situations where restoration of flow is essential and the patient is inoperable. Angioplasty is most likely to be successful when there is a clear stump of the proximal renal artery with evidence of reconstitution distally via collaterals. Extreme caution must be used when crossing a total renal occlusion, given the risk of perforation. Thrombolytic therapy has been used in a small number of patients with total occlusions.

Coexistence with Abdominal Aortic Aneurysms

It is not uncommon to find atherosclerotic renal artery stenosis in combination with an abdominal aortic aneurysm (AAA). The risks of surgical repair of an AAA are significantly increased with the additional requirement of renal bypass procedures. PTRA can be successfully performed prior to AAA repair. However, vascular access issues are clearly important. Since the *de novo* aneurysm often distorts normal anatomy and there is usually associated thrombus within the aneurysm, some interventionalists prefer the brachial approach in this patient subset. The femoral approach can be used, but extreme caution must be exercised to minimize contact with the aortic wall. If the renal artery arises within the AAA, then revascularization should be deferred to the surgeon. Or, if the renal function is normal and blood pressure is easily controlled with medications, PTRA can be performed following AAA repair. Future combinations of percutaneous stent-grafts for AAA repair with PTRA will undoubtedly be explored.

Restenotic Lesions

Lesions that have restenosed following conventional balloon angioplasty are appropriate candidates for renal artery stenting. In-stent restenosis is likely best managed by repeat balloon angioplasty. Use of a 4-cm long balloon may be preferred, to avoid the "watermelon seed" effect of balloon slippage. Caution must be exercised to avoid edge dissections, which can easily propagate into the distal renal artery. IVUS guidance for appropriate balloon sizing may be prudent in this lesion subset. Stenting within a stent can be done for circumstances where recoil is severe, however, the long-term outcome of this approach is unknown. There is currently no data for debulking strategies with directional or rotational atherectomy nor with radiation. Whatever the strategy for treating in-stent restenosis, the option of surgical intervention should remain a consideration.

Transplant Allografts

Renal graft artery stenosis occurs in 2%–10% of renal allografts.[28] This is usually manifested by uncontrolled hypertension. Renal allografts are generally placed in the pelvis, with anastamosis either to the internal or the external iliac arteries. In patients with renal allografts that have anastamosis in an end-to-end fashion to the internal iliac artery, most interventionalists choose a retrograde contralateral femoral approach. When the renal allograft is attached in and end-to-side fashion to the external iliac, a retrograde ipsilateral femoral approach is usually most appropriate. Percutaneous intervention in some renal allografts may be technically challenging, owing to the perpendicular orientation of the renal artery and difficulty in crossing the lesion with a guidewire. There remains debate as to the best treatment strategy, repeat surgery or percutaneous therapy, for transplant renal artery stenosis.[29] An individualized approach seems wise when dealing with a sole kidney. Concern has been raised that stenting the proximal portion of the renal artery will limit subsequent surgical revascularization opportunities, though this has not yet been documented to occur.

Complications

There is a considerable learning curve in the performance of PTRA and stenting.[10] Complications have been reported to occur in 5%–15% of patients, and include atheroembolization; renal artery thrombosis, dissection, or perforation; renal infarction; renal failure; subcapsular or retroperitoneal bleeding; and access site issues. Many complications can be avoided by paying exquisite attention to detail before, during, and after the procedure. A careful history and physical exam which, for example, reveals evidence of prior episodes of cholesterol embolization may alter access strategies, peri-procedural medical regimen or threshold for embarking on the procedure. Care must be taken to review diagnostic angiograms before the procedure. If adequate visualization of the renal ostium has not been achieved, further oblique views are required. It is not uncommon to find an accessory renal artery that has a previously undiagnosed critical stenosis. The most feared complication, cholesterol or atheroembolism, can be minimized by using the "no-touch" technique when instrumenting the abdominal aorta.

In a recent review of ten studies of renal artery stenting, 6 patients of the 379 total patients (1.6%) died within 10 days of stenting.[30] However, in only 2 of 379 (0.5%) was the death judged to be related to the procedure. Complications other than dialysis occurred in 42 of 379 (11%) of patients. When patients who required dialysis were added, the risk was 51 of 379 (13.5%). It is difficult in this report, however, to distinguish whether the need for dialysis was related to a procedural complication or progression of disease.

In the only published randomized trial of PTRA versus stenting, complications were similar in the two groups (10%). Complications included access site bleeding, retroperitoneal bleeding, femoral arterial pseudoaneurysm, arteriovenous fistula, renal artery dissection, renal artery thrombosis/occlusion, cholesterol embolism, and dye induced nephropathy.

Vascular Access Complications

Vascular access complications are similar to any percutaneous vascular revascularization procedure and include bleeding, pseudoaneurysm, arteriovenous fistula, retroperitoneal bleeding, thrombosis, dissection, occlusion, and infection. Most bleeding complications are related to over aggressive anticoagulation regimes, rather than sheath size. Direct fluoroscopic visualization of the guidewire as it passes into the central aorta will minimize arterial trauma and the chance of inducing a dissection.

Renal Artery Spasm

Distal vessel spasm is not infrequent and may be reduced by pretreatment with nitroglycerin or other vasodilators. Spasm occurs more frequently in younger patients with FMD, than in older individuals with ARAS.

Renal Artery Dissection/Perforation

Dissection of the renal artery may occur due to guiding catheter or guidewire trauma, during either balloon angioplasty or stenting. Excessive guide catheter manipulation at the renal ostium should be avoided. Hydrophilic guidewires are the last choice for crossing the lesion in the renal artery, due to their propensity for creating dissections and perforations. Dissections may propagate proximally or distally after PTRA or stenting. The operator must be vigilant in recognizing arterial dissections as they may lead to subsequent thrombosis and occlusion if left untreated. If a significant dissection is noted, further treatment with PTRA and additional stenting may be warranted.

Perforation through the distal renal artery into the renal parenchyma may be caused by the guidewire, with subsequent formation of a perinephric or subcapsular hematoma. The patient will typically complain of flank or abdominal pain and nausea, and hypotension and vagotonia may ensue. Evidence of an expanding perinephric hematoma may by seen on the nephrogram: initially, a location invagination will appear and the nephrogram will be less "full" than preprocedure. At later stages, the distal vascular tree will appear "compressed" or "crowded," and filling of the capillary bed will be impaired or attenuated. Heparin should be reversed with protamine and close hemodynamic monitoring is required. The patient may require urgent surgery and consultation with a vascular surgeon is advisable. Rupture of the body of the renal artery is infrequent and may occur due to balloon/stent oversizing. This complication usually requires urgent surgical repair, although covered stents may potentially be useful in this circumstance.

Renal Artery Thrombosis/Occlusion

Occlusion of the renal artery during the procedure is most often due to vessel dissection. Further treatment with balloon angioplasty and stenting may be warranted. IVUS may be useful to guide therapy in this situation. Occlusion may also be related to thrombus formation. All patients should be pretreated with aspirin prior the procedure. If the patient is allergic to aspirin, clopridogrel or ticlopidine should be substituted for aspirin. The use of intra-arterial thrombolysis for renal arterial occlusion has been reported. There is also a case report of the successful use of abcixamab and adjunctive PTRA for stent thrombosis that occurred one day after the procedure.[31] The actual incidence of subacute stent thrombosis after renal artery stenting is unknown. Some operators have extrapolated data from the coronary circulation and are recommending combination therapy with aspirin and clopidogrel after renal stenting. Future trials will hopefully shed light on this subject.

Cholesterol Emboli Syndrome

The most feared complication of percutaneous renal interventions is that of multiple cholesterol emboli syndrome. This complication is often due to excessive and aggressive catheter manipulation in a diseased abdominal aorta or iliac vessels. Cholesterol embolization may occur into the renal vascular bed or into the periphery. Warren and Vales showed that there is a threshold of embolic burden below which there are few clinical events and above which there is progressive deterioration leading to extensive thrombosis and subsequent death.[11]

Cholesterol embolization may be seen both acutely or in a delayed fashion.[12] Clinical findings include blue toes, livedo reticularis, distal extremity pain, abdominal/flank/back pain, gross hematuria, accelerated hypertension, and renal failure. Cholesterol emboli can be associated with fever, elevated erythrocyte sedimentation rate and peripheral eosinophilia. Extreme manifestations have included gangrene, nonhealing foot ulcers, spinal cord infarction, penile gangrene and hematochezia. Other delayed findings include progressive rise in the serum creatinine and persistent hypertension despite adequate angiographic revascularization. The differential diagnosis of cholesterol emboli syndrome includes polyarteritis nodosa, allergic vasculitis, and subacute bacterial endocarditis.[12] Renal failure due to cholesterol emboli syndrome may be secondary to cholesterol emboli in the renal arterioles, renal infarction, or renal tubular toxicity due to overwhelming rhabdomyolysis.[12]

Cholesterol embolization may occur spontaneously in patients with diffuse atheromatous disease. Care should be taken to screen patients for evidence of this condition prior to the procedure, as a predilection for embolization may be a relative contraindication to the planned procedure. Consideration to the use of the brachial approach should be given in patients with diffuse atheromatous disease. There is no known effective treatment for the renal manifestations of cholesterol embolization. Adequate hydration is recommended with the possible addition of sodium bicarbinate if there is severe rhabdomyolysis. There are reports of successful use of intravenous prostacyclin for the treatment of lower extremity pain and ulceration due to cholesterol emboli.

Renal Failure

Renal failure may occur as a consequence of cholesterol emboli syndrome (see above), or from the toxic effects of radiographic dye. Clearly the patient population undergoing renal artery stenting is at increased risk for dye induced nephrotoxicity due to their uderlying pathologic condition. Patients should be vigorously hydrated before, during, and after the procedure to avoid dye-related complications. Drugs with renal toxic effects should be avoided. Patients taking metformin for glucose control should preferably have the drug discontinued 48 hours before the procedure to avoid the potential complication of lactic acidosis. Metformin should not be reinstituted until a serum creatinine is checked 48 hours postprocedure. The use of Mucormist to prevent toxic effects from the contrast dye has not yet been studied for renal procedures.

Technical Complications

Balloon Rupture

Balloon rupture may occur as a consequence of a microperforation in the balloon material during hand crimping of the stent. It is also seen in the treatment of calcified lesions. Balloon rupture can be managed by forceful hand injection of contrast into the balloon lumen to partially deploy the stent. Subsequent inflations can be made with a low profile balloon within the stent.

Loss of Wire Position

If guidewire position is lost after stent deployment, the operator should take care not to pass the guidewire underneath a stent strut. Placing a large gentle curve, using a "small-radius "J-tip", or using a larger caliber wire (e.g., 0.035" Wholey) will facilitate passage through the stent away from the struts. IVUS can be used subsequently to confirm an intrastent position.

Stent Malposition

Positioning a stent too distally, if unrecognized, may increase the risk of restenosis. Even when recognized, additional (overlapping) stent deployment is required, the effect of which are unknown. A stent placed too proximally, extending into the abdominal aorta more than 2 mm will hamper future attempts at engaging the renal ostium. Diagnostic angiography in multiple oblique views may be necessary to adequately define the origin of the renal ostia to ensure proper stent positioning.

Future Directions

The results of multicenter trials of renal stenting are forthcoming. There will be further advancement in the technology such that procedures will be performed more easily and safely, through smaller guiding catheter systems. Already, premounted stents on 0.014"/0.018" balloon platforms can be advanced through 6 Fr guides. In addition, precurved braided sheaths are now available, which obviate the need for guiding catheters altogether. While these compromise the manipulability slightly, they also enable smaller arterotomy at the access site. Topics for future exploration include the utility of debulking strategies prior to stenting, the use of the cutting balloon prior to stenting, and the role of radiation therapy, coated stents, and covered stents in the renal vasculature. As technological advances make renal revascularization more feasible, the capability to distinguish which patients will truly benefit, and to what degree, will become even more critical.

References

1. Grossman W, Baim D. **Cardiac Catheterization, Angiography and Intervention**. 6th ed. Philadelphia, Williams & Wilkins, 2000:
2. Burket MW, Cooper CJ, Kennedy DJ, et al. Renal artery angioplasty and stent placement: Predictors of a favorable outcome. *Am Heart J* 2000; 139:64–71.
3. Blum U, Krumme B, Flugel P, et al. Treatment of ostial renal-artery stenoses with vascular endoprostheses after unsuccessful balloon angioplasty. *J Vasc Intervent Radiol* 1997; 8(4): 724.

4. Dorros G, Jaff M, Jain A, et al. Follow-up of primary palmaz-schatz stent placement for atherosclerotic renal artery stenosis. *Am J Cardiol* 1995; 75:1051–1055.

5. van den Ven PJG, Kaatee R, Beutler JJ. Arterial stenting and balloon angioplasty in ostial atherosclerotic renovascular disease: A randomized trial. *Lancet* 1999; 353:282–286.

6. Rocha-Singh K, Mishkel GJ, Katholi RE. Clinical predictors of improved long-term blood pressure control after successful stenting of hypertensive patients with obstructive renal artery atherosclerosis. *Cathet Cardiovasc Intervent* 1999; 47:167–172.

7. White CJ, Ramee SR, Collins TJ. Renal artery stent placement: Utility in lesions difficult to treat with balloon angioplasty. *JACC* 1997; 30:1445–1450.

8. Lim ST, Rosenfield K. Renal artery stent placement: Indications and results. *Current Science* 2000; 2:130–139.

9. Iannone LA, Underwood PL, Nath A. Effect of primary balloon expandable renal artery stents on long-term patency, renal function, and blood pressure in hypertensive and renal insufficient patients with renal artery stenosis. *Cathet Cardiovasc Diagn* 1996; 37:243–250.

10. Beek FJA, Kaatee R, Beutler JJ, et al. Complications during renal artery stent placement for atherosclerotic ostial stenosis. *Cardiovasc Inervent Radiol* 1997; 20:184–190.

11. Palmer FJ, Warren BA. Multiple cholesterol emboli syndrome complicating angiographic techniquees. *Clin Radiol* 1988; 39:519.

12. Ramos R, Cruzado JM, Palom X, et al. Cholesterol embolism associated with macroscopic renal infarction. *Nephrol Dial Transplant* 1999; 14:962–965.

13. Gruntzig A, Kuhlmann U, Lutolf U, et al. Treatment of renovascular hypertension with percutaneous transluminal dilation of a renal-artery stenosis. *Lancet* 1978; 1:801–802.

14. Tegtmeyer CJ, Dyer R, Teates CD, et al. Percutaneous transluminal dilatation of the renal arteries. *Radiology* 1980; 135:589–599.

15. Rimmer JM, Gennari FJ. Atherosclerotic renovascular disease and progressive renal failure. *Ann Intern Med* 1993; 118:712–719.

16. Dorros G, Jaff M, Mathiak L. Four-year follow-up of Palmaz-Schatz stent revascularization as treatment for atherosclerotic renal artery stenosis. *Circulation* 1998; 98:642–647.

17. Xue F, Bettmann MA, Langdon DR, et al. Outcome and cost comparison of percutaneous transluminal renal angioplasty stent placement, and renal arterial bypass grafting. *Radiology* 1999; 212(2): 378–384.

18. Cicuto KP, McLean GK, Oleaga JA, et al. Renal artery stenosis: Anatomic classification for percutaneous transluminal angioplasty. *AJR* 1981; 137:599–601.

19. Kaatee R, Beek FJA, Verschuyl EJ, et al. Atherosclerotic renal artery stenosis: Ostial or truncal. *Radiology* 1996; 199:637–640.

20. Sos TA, Pickering TG, Phil D. Percutaneous transluminal renal angioplasty in renovascular hypertension due to atheroma or fibromuscular dysplasia. *N Engl J Med* 1983; 309:274–279.

21. White CJ, Ramee SR, Collins TJ, et al. Guiding catheter-assisted renal artery angioplasty. *Cathet Cardiovasc Diagn* 1991; 23:10–13.

22. Dorros G, Prince C, Mathiak L. Stenting of a renal artery stenosis achieves better relief of the obstructive lesion than balloon angioplasty. *Cathet Cardiovasc Diagn* 1993; 29:191–198.

23. Nahman NS Jr, Maniam P, Hernandez RA Jr, et al. Renal artery pressure gradients in patients with angiographic evidence of atherosclerotic renal artery stenosis. *Am J Kid Dis* 1994; 24:695–699.

24. Rosenfield K, Losordo DW, Ramaswamy K, et al. Three-dimensional reconstruction of human coronary and peripheral arteries from images recorded during two-dimensional intravascular ultrasound examination. *Circulation* 1991; 84 (5): 1938–1956.

25. Avula S, Dorros G. Juxtaposed "kissing" stents as a technique to preserve both limbs of a bifurcating renal artery. *Cathet Cardiovasc Diagn* 1995; 36(2): 143–145.

26. Robertson IR, Barron D, Kessel D. Angioplasty through the side of a renal artery stent. *JVIR* 1998; November-December:
27. Sniderman KW, Sos TA. Percutaneous transluminal recanalization and dilatation of totally occluded renal arteries. *Radiology* 1982; 142:607–610.
28. Peregrin JH, Lacha J, Adamec M. Successful handling by stent inplantation of postoperative renal graft artery stenosis and dissection. *Nephrol Dial Transplant* 1998; 13:1004–1006.
29. Novick AC. Secondary renal vascular reconstruction for arterial disease in the native and transplant kidney. *Renal Vasc Dis Trasplant* 1994; 21:94–143.
30. Isles CG, Robertson S, Hill D. Management of renovascular disease: A review of renal artery stenting in ten studies. *Q J Med* 1999; 92:159–167.
31. Berkompas DC. Abciximab combined with angioplasty in a patient with renal artery stent subacute thrombosis. *Cathet Cardiovasc Diagn* 1998; 45:272–274.

6

What Are the Technical and Clinical Results of Renal Artery Stenting?

Mark C. Bates, MD, FACC

Introduction

The long-term clinical sequelae of renal artery stenosis have been detailed in several natural history studies.[1–7] Attempts at improving outcome with medical therapy have been disappointing, and surgical revascularization, although effective and durable, has a high risk of perioperative complication limiting its utility.[8–14] The peremptory challenge in evaluating renal artery stenting as a new endovascular treatment strategy for this frequently silent disease is to first prove the procedure can be performed with a high degree of technical success and low risk of complication. A detailed review of the current literature on early outcomes following renal stenting, including observations from our center, is to follow. This chapter also provides unique insight into historical issues and technical advances that have positively affected the technical success of renal stent supported angioplasty.

History

Many of the interventional techniques that have allowed progress in the field of renal artery stenting should be credited to the early pioneers who performed "stand-alone" renal angioplasty.

The material in this chapter was sponsored by Camcare Research Institute, Charleston Area Medical Center, Charleston, WV and Robert C. Byrd Health Sciences Center, West Virginia University School of Medicine Division, Charleston, WV

From Jaff MR (ed): *Endovascular Therapy for Atherosclerotic Renal Artery Stenosis: Present and Future.* Armonk, NY: Future Publishing Co, Inc.; ©2001.

Andreas Grüntzig reported the first renal artery balloon angioplasty in 1978 and work in the following decade by Tegtmeyer, Sos, Martin and others set the stage for providing very important developments in catheter design that have allowed us now to enjoy the current technical results reported in this chapter.[15-18] Alternatives to balloon angioplasty were considered as the early enthusiasm regarding renal artery angioplasty was tempered by concerns about the durability of the procedure. The high risk of recurrence in these patients was a recurrent theme throughout the medical literature in the mid-to-late 1980s. The frequent association of dense calcification and common ostial location of these lesions, resulted in early recoil related lumen loss amplifying the restenosis process.[16,19,20] The concept of providing scaffolding via an endovascular prosthesis or stent renewed interest in transcatheter intervention for renal artery stenosis in the 1990s.

The first generation stents were slotted tube designs lending to their inherit rigidity adversely affecting the deployment characteristics. The pausity of available guide catheters and stents designed specifically for placement in the renal artery led to innovative techniques like the transbrachial approach described by Dr. Dorros[21] and several transfemoral techniques.[22,23]

Throughout the country in the early 1990s, high volume operators developed their own techniques for stent placement and it was only in the last few months that more flexible stents and stent delivery systems specifically designed for renal stent placement became available in the United States. The following description of the early clinical outcomes of stent supported renal angioplasty include complications and technical limitations of an evolving art.

Learning Curve

Understanding the learning curve of any new procedure is germane to the discussion of clinical and technical outcomes. Operator experience has been shown to increase technical success in renal angioplasty and is an important variable in interpretation of clinical experience with renal stents.[24,25] The number of percutaneous transluminal renal stent procedures that are necessary to ensure operator safety and minimize complications have not been clearly defined.

In our series of over 500 renal stent patients we noted progressive decrease in mortality and increased technical success with experience (Figure 1). Rosha-Singh showed similar findings observing no deaths in the last one hundred patients in that two hundred patient series.[26]

Interestingly, these observations on the learning curve for renal stenting are very similar to those described by Martin for "stand alone" balloon renal angioplasty.[27]

We estimate that 100 transcatheter renal angioplasty procedures should be done at a single center before attempting complex transcatheter interventions in patients with solitary kidneys or hostile aortas. This is important information when digesting the results of several renal stent studies since many have small numbers of patients.

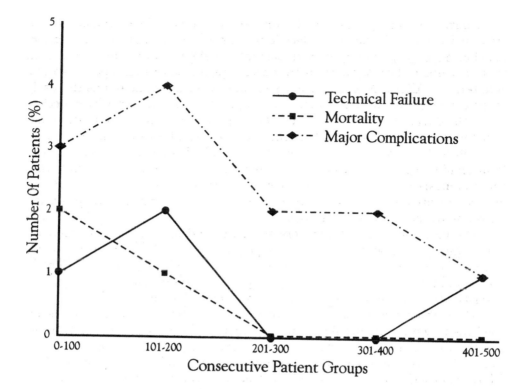

Figure 1. *Single operator mortality and morbidity observations over 7 years.* Technical failure defined as inability to deploy stent, residual stenosis > 30%, and/or persistent gradient. Major complications defined as pseudoaneurysm, bleeding requiring transfusion, retroperitoneal bleed, acute renal failure, cholesterol embolization, ischemic bowel. Mortality details; Patient 1-atheroemboli-bowel infarction complicated by sepsis-death, Patient 2 – heparin induced thrombocytopenia with retroperitoneal bleed and death related to shock, Patient 3 – pneumonia-sepsis in 86-year-old woman.

Lessons Learned

A retrospective review of factors that have improved early technical results at our institution suggests; operator experience, improvement of equipment/technique and patient selection are important factors. Specific "lessons learned" based on anecdotal experiences are somewhat subjective, but important to note:

1. Early in the series, a patient developed atheroembolic disease to the small bowel resulting in acute ischemic bowel and infarction. Cautious manipulation of diagnostic or guide catheters in the abdominal aorta below the diaphragm is prudent. Any time catheter manipulation is needed in this region, the catheter is stationed posteriorly as it is retracted avoiding interaction with the anterior situated mesenteric vessels.

2. The transfemoral technique we now utilize occasionally requires crossing the lesion with the guide catheter over a balloon. A guide catheter with side holes allows continuous renal perfusion during balloon/stent exchanges and may reduce renal ischemia time.

3. Minimizing contrast dosage is important. A low dose contrast diagnostic angiogram is done to confirm the co-axial alignment prior to guide catheter placement. We arbitrarily try to use less than 50 cc or 20 cc of contrast in patients with normal creatinine or elevated creatinine respectively reducing the risks of post procedural contrast induced azotemia.

4. The first 88 patients in our series were all done via brachial access. We now reserve transbrachial approach for patients with tortuous "hostile aortas," severe aortoiliac disease or as Sos described those patients with severe inferior angulation of the renal artery.[16] This has reduced access complications.

5. Three-dimensional computed tomography (CT) scans have taught us a lot about renal artery anatomy (Figure 2). Verschuyl et al. reviewed 200 CT scans and found the left and right renal artery ostium are generally seen best in a 20 degrees left anterior oblique view.[28] However, extremes of posterior and anterior origin for both kidneys were noted. We have made similar observations from MRA and frequently use the renal MRA when available to calculate obliquity of the image intensifier prior to contrast injection (Figures 3a and 3b). Precise C-arm angulation im-

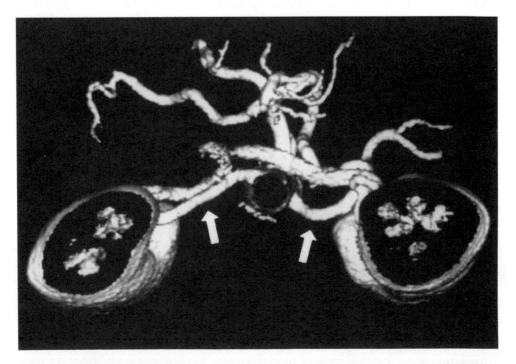

Figure 2. Three-dimensional CT-scan of normal renal arteries (arrows) demonstrating typical posterior take off of left renal artery.

proves accuracy of stent placement, especially when treating an ostial lesion (Figures 3c and 3d).

6. Using the no-touch technique described by Feldman, et al. in patients with hostile aortas or approaching those patients from a brachial approach, we believe has reduced the risk of embolization and/or ostial guide catheter trauma.[29]

7. Meticulous hemodynamic monitoring is an imperative on engaging the renal artery with any catheter since damping is a cardinal marker of engagement into soft plaque. With this technique we do not see contrast staining in the aorta in patients with medial necrosis or aneurysmal disease thus avoiding hydrolic injury to the renal ostium or aorta during injection.

Technical Success

Technical success as defined by minimal residual luminal encroachment and successful stent deployment without *immediate* periprocedural major complication can be achieved in most patients (95–100%) (Table 1).[22,25,26,30–45] The technical success in our large series of patients suggests almost all patients irrespective of their anatomy can now be treated with stent supported renal angioplasty (Figure 1). Initial failures were related to difficulty in crossing the lesion or tracking the stent via brachial approach and/or adequate guide support from a transfemoral approach.

Clinical Results

The long-term outcome of renal artery stenting is described elsewhere in this monograph. The immediate in-hospital clinical findings following renal artery angioplasty and stent placement are of questionable long-term clinical importance. Frequently, antihypertensive drugs are held at the time of renal artery stent placement and therefore, the following morning's analysis of blood pressure as a predischarge clinical endpoint is very confusing. Also, stenting of critical renal artery disease is frequently followed by spontaneous diuresis, indirectly affecting early blood pressure results. Most authors recognize the limitation of early blood pressure analysis and for that reason do not include this data in the study.

Likewise, initial results in creatinine and blood urea nitrogen (BUN) are confounded by the frequent use of postprocedural hydration. We observed a statistically significant improvement in overall creatinine in our series (n = 508 pre-Cr 1.57, post 1.40, $p < 0.05$) when preprocedure values were compared to Cr at discharge. The difference was no longer significant at 1 month, suggesting periprocedural variables like hydration may have falsely lowered the discharge creatinine. In our experience, elevation in the creatinine immediately following the procedure is most likely related to contrast induced nephropathy with a secondary bimodal jump in creatinine 72 hours following the procedure most likely related to atheroembolization.

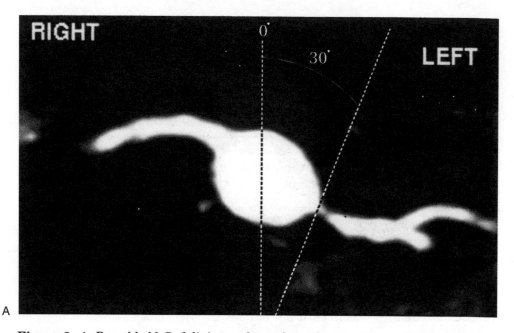

Figure 3. A. Breathhold Gadolinium enhanced renal magnetic resonance angiogram (MRA). Note left renal stenosis and slight posterior origin.

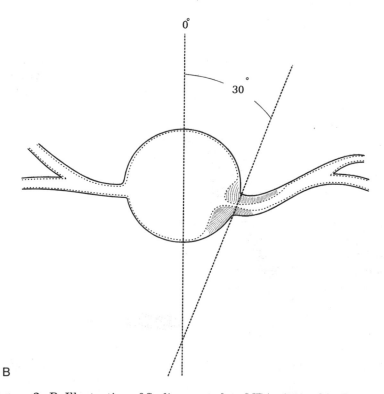

Figure 3. B. Illustration of findings noted on MRA pictured in Figure 3A.

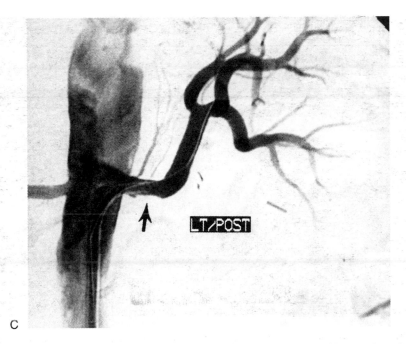

C

Figure 3. C. Angiogram of lesion viewed at 30° LAO based on MRA angle calculation depicted in Figure 3A.

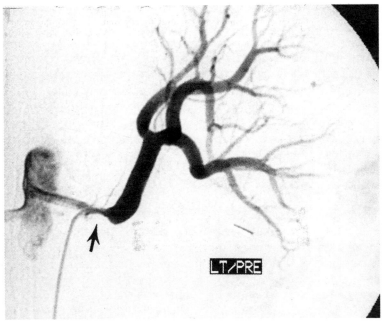

D

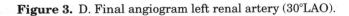

Figure 3. D. Final angiogram left renal artery (30°LAO).

Table 1.

Literature Review of Renal Stent Studies Detailing Technical Success and Mortality/Major Complications.

Study (ref)	Year	No. Pts.	Tech Success	Mortality	Major Complications
Rees (30)	1991	28	96%	3.6%	7.0%
Joffre (31)	1992	21	100%	0.0%	4.8%
Raynaud (22)	1994	15	100%	0.0%	6.7%
McLeod (32)	1995	29	100%	3.4%	13.8%
Iannoure (33)	1996	63	99%	14.2%	33.0%
Rundback (34)	1996	20	96%	0.0%	5.0%
Harjai (35)	1997	66	100%	0.0%	0.0%
Blum (36)	1997	68	100%	0.0%	4.4%
Taylor (24)	1997	29	100%	3.5%	24.0%
Harden (37)	1997	32	100%	3.0%	0.0%
Boisclair (25)	1997	33	100%	0.0%	21.0%
White (38)	1997	100	99%	1.0%	2.0%
Dorros (39)	1998	163	99%	1.8%	1.0%
Gross (40)	1998	30	100%	3.0%	0.0%
Fiala (41)	1998	21	95%	0.0%	19.0%
Tuttle (42)	1998	129	98%	3.0%	4.1%
Henry, M (43)	1999	210	99%	0.5%	1.2%
van de Ven (44)	1998	28	85%	0.0%	0.0%
Rosha Singh (26)	1999	150	97.3%	1.3%	2.6%
Rodriguez-Lupez (45)	1999	108	97.6%	3.7%	7.2%

Note: Definition of major complications varied and included acute renal failure, myocardial infarction, transfusions, retroperitoneal bleed, and renal perforation. Ref = reference, N = number of patients in each study, technical success = successful stent placement without significant residual stenosis.

Elevation of the creatinine following the procedure was extremely uncommon in the patients with preprocedural normal creatinine, but the most common cause of prolonged hospital stay in patients with baseline azotemia.

The second most common cause overall of prolonged hospital stay in our series was access complication. Analysis of the data base for early predismissal clinical markers of long-term durability or outcome is currently underway.

Discussion

Transcatheter options for renal artery stenosis have changed dramatically since the "dilatation catheter with tipped distensible sausage shape balloon segment" was used by Grüntzig to perform the first reported renal angioplasty over 20 years ago.[15] Just as balloons and guiding catheters have dramatically improved since inception we expect continued evolution and improvement in stent design and delivery systems for renal artery stenosis.

Currently, there are no stent platforms or delivery systems specifically designed for renal intervention. Innovative techniques by pioneers in the field have shown that even in the absence of dedicated catheter designs a stent can be placed in the renal artery ostium with a technical success of > 97% and early clinical success of > 95%. Undoubtedly, as the art progresses we can expect to see improvement in technical results and perhaps better clinical outcomes.

The lower morbidity and mortality of stent supported angioplasty compared to surgery and high technical success could allow renal artery stenting to become the gold standard for renal revascularization assuming durability data confirms long term patency and clinical benefit. As renal artery stenting matures, and complications diminish, there will be increasing utilization of stents for atherosclerotic renal artery disease.

References

1. Wollenweber J, Sheps SG, David DG. Clinical course of atherosclerotic renovascular disease. *Am J Cardiol* 1968; 21:60–71.
2. Stewart BH, Dustan HP, Kiser WS, et al. Correlation of angiography and natural history in evaluation of patients with renovascular hypertension. *J Urol* 1970; 104:231–238.
3. Schreiber MJ, Pohl MA, Novick AC. The natural history of atherosclerotic and fibrous renal artery disease. *Urol Clin North Am* 1984; 11:383–392.
4. Zucchelli P, Chiarini C, Zuccala A, Delgi Espositi E. Renal ischemic is the real problem in renovascular hypertension in Gloriosos N (ed): **Renovascular Hypertension**. New York: Raven Press, 1987, pp 273–278.
5. Tollefson DE, Ernst CB. Natural history of atherosclerotic renal artery stenosis associated with aortic disease. *J Vasc Surg* 1991; 14:327–331.
6. Zierler RE, Bergelin RO, Isaacson JA, et al. Natural history of renal artery stenosis: A prospective study with duplex ultrasound. *J Vasc Surg* 1994; 19:250–258.
7. Strandness DE. Natural history of renal artery stenosis. *Am J Kid Dis* 1994; 24:630–635.
8. Lawrie GM, Morris GC, Glaeser DH, et al. Renovascular reconstruction: Factors affecting long-term prognosis in 919 patients followed up to 31 years. *Am J Cardiol* 1989; 63:1085–1092.
9. Novick AC, Ziegelbaum M, Vidt DG, et al. Trends in surgical revascularization for renal artery disease. *JAMA* 1987; 257:498–501.
10. Franklin SS, Young JD, Maxwell MH, et al. Operative morbidity and mortality in renovascular disease. *JAMA* 1975; 231:1148–1153.
11. Foster JH, Maxwell MJ, Franklin SS, et al. Renovascular occlusive disease: Results of operative treatment. *JAMA* 1975; 231:1043–1048.
12. Lankford NS, Donohue JP, Grim CE, et al. Results of surgical treatment of renovascular hypertension. *J Urol* 1979; 122:439–441.
13. Ying CY, Tifft CP, Gavras H, et al. Renal revascularization in the azotemic hypertensive patient resistant to therapy. *N Engl J Med* 1984; 311:1070–1075.
14. Hansen KJ, Starr SM, Sands E, et al. Contemporary surgical management of renovascular disease. *J Vasc Surg* 1992; 16:319–331.
15. Grüntzig A, Vetter W, Meier B, et al. Treatment of renovascular hypertension with percutaneous transluminal dilatation of a renal-artery stenosis. *Lancet* 1978; 1:801–802.
16. Sos TA, Pickering TG, Phil D, et al. Percutaneous transluminal renal angioplasty in renovascular hypertension due to atheroma or fibromuscular dysplasia. *N Engl J Med* 1983; 309:274–279.
17. Tegtmeyer CJ, Sos TA. Techniques of renal angioplasty. *Radiology* 1986; 161:577–586.
18. Martin LG, Cork RD, Kaufman SL. Long-term results of angioplasty in 110 patients with renal artery stenosis. *JVIR* 1992; 3:619–626.
19. Plouin PF, Darne B, Chatellier G. Restenosis after a first percutaneous transluminal renal angioplasty. *Hypertension* 1993; 21:89–96.

20. Dean RH, Callis JT, Smith BM, et al. Failed percutaneous transluminal renal angioplasty: Experience with lesions requiring operative intervention. *J Vasc Surg* 1987; 6:301–307.
21. Avula S, Dorros G. Juxtaposed "kissing" stents as a technique to preserve both limbs if a balloon angioplasty. *N Engl J Med* 1997; 336(7): 459–465.
22. Raynaud AC, Beyssen BM, Turmel-Rodrigues LE, et al. Renal artery stent placement: Immediate and midterm technical and clinical results. *J Vasc Interv Radiol* 1994; 5(6): 849–858.
23. Saeed M. Aortoiliac and renal artery stenting. Handbook of Interventional Radiologic Procedures, 2nd ed. Boston: Little, Brown: 1996; pp.103–114.
24. Taylor A, Sheppard D, Macleod MJ, et al. Renal artery stent placement in renal artery stenosis: Technical and early clinical results. *Clin Radiol* 1997; 52(6): 451–457.
25. Boisclair C, Therasse E, Oliva VL, et al. Treatment of renal angioplasty failure by percutaneous renal artery stenting with Palmaz stents: Midterm technical and clinical results. *Am J Roentgenol* 1997; 168(1): 245–251.
26. Rocha-Singh KJ, Mishkel GJ, Katholi RE, et al. Clinical predictors of improved long-term blood pressure control after successful stenting of hypertensive patients with obstructive renal artery atherosclerosis. *Cathet Cardiovasc Intervent* 1999; 47:167–172.
27. Martin LG, Casarella WJ, Spaugh JP, et al. Renal artery angioplasty: Increased technical success and decreased complications in the second 100 patients. *Radiology* 1986; 159(3): 631–634.
28. Verschuyl EJ, Kaatee R, Beek FJA, et al. Renal artery origins: Best angiographic projection angles. *Radiology* 1997; 205:115–120.
29. Feldman RL, Wargovich TJ, Bittl JA. No-touch technique for reducing aortic wall trauma during renal artery stenting. *Cathet Cardiovasc Intervent* 1999; 46:245–248.
30. Rees CR, Palmaz JC, Becker GJ, et al. Palmaz stent in atherosclerotic stenoses involving the ostia of the renal arteries: Preliminary report of a multicenter study. *Radiology* 1991; 181(2): 507–514.
31. Joffre F, Rousseau H, Bernadet P, et al. Midterm results of renal artery stenting. *Cardiovasc Intervent Radiol* 1992; 15(5): 313–318.
32. MacLeod M, Taylor AD, Baxter G, et al. Renal artery stenosis managed by Palmaz stent insertion: Technical and clinical outcome. *J Hypertens* 1995; 13:1791–1795.
33. Iannone LA, Underwood PL, Nath A, et al. Effect of primary balloon expandable renal artery stents on long-term patency, renal function, and blood pressure in hypertensive and renal insufficient patients with renal artery stenosis. *Cathet Cardiovasc Diagn* 1996; 37(3): 243–250.
34. Rundback JH, Jacobs JM. Percutaneous renal artery stent placement for hypertension and azotemia: Pilot study. *Am J Kidney Dis* 1996; 28(2): 214–219.
35. Harjai K, Shosla S, Shaw D, et al. Effect of gender on outcomes following renal artery stent placement for renovascular hypertension. *Cathet Cardiovasc Diagn* 1997; 42:381–386.
36. Joffre FG, Rousseau HP, Aziza R, et al. Renal artery stent placement: Long-term results with the Wallstent Endoprosthesis. *Radiology* 1994; 191:713–719.
37. Harden PN, MacLeod MJ, Rodger RS, et al. Effect of renal-artery stenting on progression of renovascular renal failure. *Lancet* 1997; 349(9059): 1133–1136.
38. White CJ, Ramee SR, Collins TJ, et al. Renal artery stent placement: Utility in lesions difficult to treat with balloon angioplasty. *J Am Coll Cardiol* 1997; 30(6): 1445–1450.
39. Dorros G, Jaff M, Mathiak L, et al. Four-year follow up of Palmaz-Schatz stent revascularization as treatment for atherosclerotic renal artery stenosis. *Circulation* 1998; 98:642–647.
40. Gross CM, Krämer J, Waigland J, et al. Ostial renal artery stent placement for atherosclerotic renal artery stenosis in patients with coronary artery disease. *Cathet Cardiovasc Diagn* 1998; 45:1–8.

41. Fiala LA, Jackson MR, Gillespie DL, et al. Primary stenting of atherosclerotic renal artery ostial stenosis. *Ann Vasc Surg* 1998; 12(2): 128–133.
42. Tuttle KR, Chouinard RF, Webber JT, et al. Treatment of atherosclerotic ostial renal artery stenosis with the intravascular stent. *Am J Kid Dis* 1998; 32(4): 611–622.
43. Henry M, Amor M, Henry I, et al. Stents in the treatment of renal artery stenosis: Long-term follow-up. *J Endovasc Surg* 1999; 6(1): 42–51.
44. Van de Ven PJG, Beutler JJ, Kaatee R, et al. Transluminal vascular stent for ostial atherosclerotic renal artery stenosis. *Lancet* 1995; 346:672–674.
45. Rodriquez-Lopez JA, Werner A, Ray LI, et al. Renal artery stenosis treated with stent deployment: Indications, technique, and outcome for 108 patients. *J Vasc Surg* 1999; 29(4): 617–624.

7

The Role for Renal Intervention in "Flash" Pulmonary Edema and Unstable Angina

Christopher J. White, MD and Stephen R. Ramee, MD

Introduction

The physiologic effects of renal artery stenosis (RAS) depend on the presence or absence of a normally functioning contralateral renal artery.[1] Patients with significant unilateral RAS generally manifest vasoconstrictor mediated hypertension. In this model, the underperfused kidney secretes renin which stimulates production of angiotensin, an extremely potent vasconstrictor, and aldosterone which promotes sodium and water retention. The normally functioning contralateral kidney responds to the volume overload secondary to aldosterone with a natiuresis. This natiuresis prevents volume overload from occurring but leads to continued stimulation of renin and angiotensin resulting in a sustained, and often severe systemic hypertension.

Patients with bilateral RAS or those with a solitary kidney and a stenotic renal artery (functional bilateral RAS), manifest volume-dependent hypertension. These patients lack a normal kidney for natiuresis, and the subsequent volume overload suppresses the renin angiotensin system. This results in a volume overload state with can lead to sustained hypertension and decompensated congestive heart failure. It has been reported that approximately one-quarter of patients with atherosclerotic renal artery disease will suffer pulmonary edema.[2] Other factors contributing to cardiac decompensation in

From Jaff MR (ed): *Endovascular Therapy for Atherosclerotic Renal Artery Stenosis: Present and Future*. Armonk, NY: Future Publishing Co, Inc.; ©2001.

patients with stable angina and chronic congestive heart failure (CHF) include volume overload secondary to renal insufficiency, and depressed systolic function.

Progression or worsening of renovascular hypertension may also precipitate clinical instability in a patient with chronic coronary ischemia. Patients with stable coronary lesions may decompensate due to uncontrolled hypertension of renovascular hypertension. The increased myocardial oxygen consumption due to the elevated blood pressure (afterload) often responds favorably to renal revascularization.[3]

Background

Atherosclerotic RAS is the most common, though infrequent (< 5%), cause of secondary hypertension in the general hypertensive population. However, in the population of patients with hypertension and atherosclerosis, the incidence of RAS is increased.[4] This is particularly true for patients with uncontrolled hypertension and coronary disease or known peripheral vascular disease where the incidence varies between 20% and 33%. In patients undergoing coronary angiography for suspected coronary artery disease, the incidence of RAS ranges from 15% to 18%.[5–8] In patients with known aneurysmal or occlusive peripheral vascular disease, one study demonstrated associated RAS in 28%.[9] In patients with renal insufficiency the incidence of unsuspected RAS was 24%.[2]

A recent study from Wake Forest University School of Medicine, addressed the issue of the pathogenesis of pulmonary edema associated with hypertension. They studied 38 patients with acute and follow-up echocardiography. Interestingly, they found that the left ventricular function was usually well preserved with normal systolic wall motion in these subjects. There was no evidence of severe mitral regurgitation during any acute episode. They concluded that acute pulmonary edema was most likely the result of diastolic dysfunction in this group of patients.[10]

In a series of 55 consecutive patients with renovascular hypertension and renal failure (serum creatinine > 142 μmol/L), Pickering and coworkers tried to determine contributing factors in 13 patients who presented with pulmonary edema.[2] Bilateral RAS and the presence of coronary disease were each independently associated with the occurrence of pulmonary edema. Pulmonary edema was more common in patients with bilateral RAS (92% vs. 65%, p < 0.001), or if coronary artery disease was present (62% vs. 24%, p < 0.025).

Percutaneous Intervention

Over an 18-month period, we treated 48 patients with RAS (> 70% diameter stenosis) and medically refractory hypertension, defined as blood pressure greater than 140/90 mmHg on three or more medications.[11] The patients received balloon expandable Palmaz (Cordis, Miami, FL) stents from either a brachial or femoral access site, and were part of a prospective registry. The chief complaint in 40% (n = 20) was unstable angina pectoris (UAP), and in

60% (n = 28) decompensated CHF (pulmonary edema). Two-thirds of all patients had bilateral RAS (UAP = 60%, CHF = 72%). All of the UAP patients and 86% of the CHF patients had significant (> 70% diameter stenosis) coronary artery disease. The patients were divided into subgroups based upon whether or not they received coronary intervention (PTCA) in addition to the renal stent placement. The decision regarding the performance of PTCA was left to the operator's discretion. The majority of patients who did not receive PTCA had diffuse coronary disease not amenable to PTCA.

The 20 patients with UAP were divided into those undergoing PTCA (n = 13) and those without PTCA (n = 7). The groups were similar in their baseline characteristics including age, left ventricular ejection fraction, presence of significant coronary disease, and Canadian Cardiovascular Society angina class (Table 1). Bilateral RAS was present in 60%. At 24 hours there was improvement of at least one CCS angina class in 90% of the 20 UAP patients treated (Figure 1). There was also significant improvement in both the systolic and diastolic blood pressure compared to baseline (Figure 2). There was no change in renal function.

At 6-month follow-up, one patient had died and one patient did not return for follow-up. Of the 18 remaining patients, 72% maintained the clinical benefit with a persistent benefit in their CCS class. There continued to be a significant improvement in blood pressure control and no significant change in renal function. Patients were stratified for outcome by the performance of renal stent with coronary revascularization with PTCA versus only renal artery stent placement (Figure 3). Interestingly, there was no difference in outcomes between the groups suggesting that the dominant benefit received was the renal intervention.

The 28 patients with CHF and pulmonary edema undergoing renal artery stent placement were also divided into those with concomitant PTCA (n = 6) and those without PTCA (n = 22). The two groups had similar baseline characteristics with the exception that the left ventricular ejection fraction was higher in the group that received PTCA (Table 2). Bilateral RAS

Table 1.

Unstable Angina Baseline Patient Characteristics Stratified by Treatment with or without PTCA.[11]

UAP Group	PTCA (+) (n = 13)	PTCA (−) (n = 7)
Age	66 ± 14	69 ± 10
LVEF	59 ± 12	55 ± 15
CAD (≥ 70%)	13 (100%)	7 (100%)
CCS class (1–4)	3.1 ± 0.8	3.1 ± 0.7

UAP = unstable angina pectoris, LVEF = left ventricular ejection fraction, CAD = coronary artery disease, CCS = Canadian Cardiovascular Society, PTCA = percutaneous transluminal coronary angioplasty.

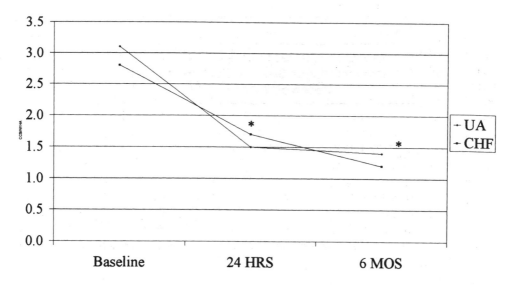

Figure 1. Acute and chronic results of renal stents in UA and CHF patients. CCS = Candian Cardiovascular Society, NYHA = New York Heart Association, UA = unstable angina (n = 20), CHF = congestive heart failure (n = 28). *p < 0.05 compared to baseline.[11]

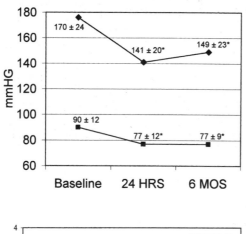

Figure 2. UAP group's blood pressure response. *p = < 0.05 compared to baseline.[11]

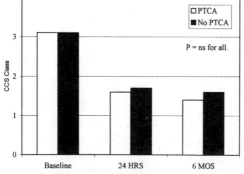

Figure 3. Effect of renal stent placement with or without PTCA in patients with UAP (n = 20) on CCS angina class.[11]

Table 2.

Congestive Heart Failure Baseline Patient Characteristics Stratified by Whether they Received PTCA or Not.[11]

CHF Group	PTCA (+) (n = 6)	PTCA (–) (n = 22)
Age	72 ± 9	66 ± 9
LVEF	46 ± 20	28 ± 4*
CAD (≥ 70%)	6 (100%)	18 (82%)
NYHA class (I–IV)	3.1 ± 0.9	2.7 ± 0.9

CHF = congestive heart failure, LVEF = left ventricular ejection fraction, CAD = coronary artery disease, NYHA = New York Heart Association, PTCA = percutaneous transluminal coronary angioplasty. *P = 0.04.

was present in 72% of the CHF patients. At 24 hours there was improvement of at least one NHYA class in 86% of the 28 CHF patients treated (Figure 1). There was a significant improvement in both the systolic and diastolic blood pressure compared to baseline (Figure 4). There was no change in renal function.

At 6-month follow-up, five patients had died and one patient did not return for follow-up. Of the 22 patients remaining, 73% maintained the clinical benefit with a persistent improvement in NYHA class (Figure 1). There continued to be a significant improvement in blood pressure control and no change in renal function. When the patients were stratified for outcome regarding the performance of coronary revascularization with PTCA, interestingly, there was no difference (Figure 5).

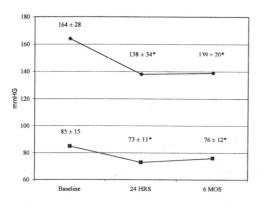

Figure 4. Congestive heart failure group's blood pressure response. *p = < 0.05 compared to baseline.[11]

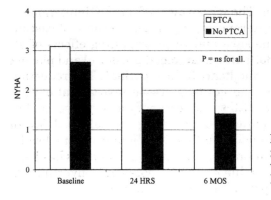

Figure 5. Effect of renal stent placement with or without PTCA in patients with congestive heart failure (n = 28) on NYHA class.[11]

Surgery

Messina and coworkers reported the outcome of surgical revascularization in 17 patients with volume dependent renovascular hypertension and bilateral RAS.[12] Pulmonary edema occurred despite a normal left ventricular ejection fraction in 65%. Bilateral disease was present in 94% and an occluded renal artery was present in 54%. A variety of surgical approaches was selected including bypass, endarterectomy, and angioplasty in one patient. Contralateral nephrectomy was performed in 41% and concomitant aortic reconstruction was performed in 24%.

They reported excellent results for surgical revascularization. Two of the three patients requiring dialysis before surgery were able to function without dialysis. After approximately 2 years of follow-up, one (6%) patient's hypertension was cured, and improvement was noted in 16 (94%). Only one patient had recurrence of pulmonary edema during follow-up. The authors urged that in occluded renal arteries ≥ 7 cm in length every attempt be made to revascularize the kidney before nephrectomy is considered. The authors emphasized the common factors among patients presenting with pulmonary edema and renovascular hypertension including bilateral RAS, left ventricular hypertrophy, renal insufficiency and uncontrolled hypertension.

Summary

The pathophysiology of RAS is complex and depends on the many variables. Stimulation of the renin angiotensin aldosterone cascade results in volume overload in patients with bilateral RAS and vasoconstriction in patients with unilateral disease. Both volume overload and vasconstriction cause significant decompensation in patients with ischemic heart disease and congestive heart failure. It is not difficult to postulate a scenario in which a patient with compensated heart failure is adversely effected by bilateral RAS. The increased afterload secondary to the vasocontriction results in increased myocardial oxygen demand which may result in decompensation of the stable angina patient.

Relief of the RAS by stenting removes the stimulus for renin production with normalization of renal perfusion. The withdrawal of renin stimulation reduces angiotensin secretion and aldosterone secretion. The absence of vasconstrictor effects of angiotensin and the salt- and water-retaining effects of aldosterone result in clinical benefit. Both afterload (blood pressure) and plasma volume decrease, helping to stabilize the heart failure patient. The reduction in blood pressure (afterload) and preload act to decrease myocardial oxygen consumption, which benefits patients with severe coronary artery disease. Renal stent placement also helps these patients by restoring normal blood flow to the kidney resulting in natiuresis (in addition to lowering aldosterone levels) which prevents volume overload. Additionally, once the renal stenosis has been treated, these patients can then receive life-saving angiotensin converting enzyme inhibitor medications without precipitating renal failure.

References

1. Simon N, Franklin SS, Bleifer KH, et al. Clinical characteristics of renovascular hypertension. *J Am Med Assoc* 1972; 220:1209–1218.
2. Pickering TG, Devereux RB, James GD, et al. Recurrent pulmonary edema in hypertension due to bilateral renal artery stenosis: Treatment by angioplasty or surgical revacularisation. *Lancet* 1988; Sept: 551–552.
3. Tami LF, McElderry MW, Al-Adli, et al. Renal artery stenosis presenting as crescendo angina pectoris. *Cath Cardiovasc Diag* 1995; 35:252–256.
4. Jacobsen HR. Ischemic renal disease: An overlooked clinical entity? *Kidney Int* 1988; 34:729–743.
5. Eyler WR, Clark GJ, Rian RL, et al. Angiography of the renal areas including a comparative study of renal arterial stenosis with and without hypertension. *Radiology* 1962; 78:879–892.
6. Jean WJ, Al-Bittar I, Xwicke DL, et al. High incidence of renal artery stenosis in patients with coronary artery disease. *Cathet Cardiovasc Diagn* 1994; 32:8–10.
7. Olin JW, Melia M, Young JR, et al. Prevalence of atherosclerosis renal artery stenosis in patients with atherosclerosis elsewhere. *Am J Med* 1990; 88:46N–51N.
8. Harding MB, Smith LR, Himmelstein SI, et al. Renal artery stenosis: Prevalence and associated risk factors in patients undergoing routine cardiac catheterization. *J Am Soc Nephrol* 1992; 2:1608–1616.
9. Valentine RJ, Clagett GP, Miller GL, et al. The coronary risk of unsuspected renal artery stenosis. *J Vasc Surg* 1993; 18:433–440.
10. Gandhi SK, Powers JC, Nomeir AM, et al. The pathogenesis of acute pulmonary edema associated with hypertension. *N Engl J Med* 2001; 344:17–22.
11. Khosla S, White CJ, Collins TJ, et al. Effects of renal artery stent implantation in patients with renovascular hypertension presenting with unstable angina or congestive heart failure. *Am J Cardiol* 1997; 80(3): 363–366.
12. Messina LM, Zelenock GB, Yao KA, et al. Renal revascularization for recurrent pulmonary edema in patients with poorly controlled hypertension and renal insufficiency: A distinct subgroup of patients with arteriosclerotic renal artery occlusive disease. *J Vasc Surg* 1992; 15:73–82.

8

Renal Artery Stenting Versus Surgery:

Which is the Optimal Therapy for Atherosclerotic Renal Artery Stenosis in the New Millennium

Richard P. Cambria, MD and John L. Kaufman, MD

Introduction

Over the past two decades, there has been an explosion in both knowledge and sophistication in management strategies for patients with pressure reducing lesions of the main renal artery. Specific medical therapy at two points on the renin angiotensin cascade in the form of angiotensin converting enzyme inhibitors, and more recently, specific angiotension receptor blockers have both revolutionized the medical management of renovascular hypertension, and provided important components of the medical management of such diverse problems as chronic left heart failure and diabetic nephropathy. The present chapter focuses on the contemporary evolution of the variety of mechanical interventions to correct renal artery stenosis and/or occlusion. The focus is on specific judgmental and technical considerations from the perspective of a treating vascular surgeon and/or interventionalist.

While it has been known for some time that renal artery occlusive lesions can mediate a severe form of hypertension, often refractory to medical therapy, only recently has attention been focused on renovascular disease as a cause of

From Jaff MR (ed): *Endovascular Therapy for Atherosclerotic Renal Artery Stenosis: Present and Future*. Armonk, NY: Future Publishing Co, Inc.;©2001.

renal excretory dysfunction, possibly leading to end stage renal disease and the need for renal replacement therapy.[1] In contemporary practice, sufficient attention has been focused on the latter consideration, that pleas are being made for more aggressive diagnosis and therapy (in particular, with endovascular techniques) of a disease process where there are still considerable gaps in knowledge with respect to the indications for interventions, the natural history of the lesions and the patients, and in particular, in predicting the functional response of revascularization when the goal of intervention is preservation of renal function.

Atherosclerotic renovascular disease (RVD), which accounts for more than 90% of patients presenting for treatment in contemporary practice, occurs in a population of patients with demographic and clinical features typical of patients with diffuse atherosclerosis. Displayed in Table 1 are demographic and clinical features in a group of nearly 300 patients treated at our institution for RVD during the interval 1976–1991. Note that 50% of our patients had some degree of renal excretory dysfunction, almost 30% had but a single functioning kidney; in 60% of these patients, the indication for intervention was at least, in part, renal function salvage. Furthermore, the frequently associated coronary artery disease introduces the potential for both significant perioperative morbidity and limitation on life expectancy. RVD is an important marker for associated coronary disease and this association occurs in a quantitative fashion, i.e., more severe degrees of renal artery stenosis and/or occlusion are associated with more anatomically severe coronary disease.[2] Parallel data are available from our own experience in patients undergoing combined aortic and renal artery reconstruction as opposed to isolated aortic reconstruction. Displayed in Table 2 are variables referable to associated coronary disease in a cohort of patients who underwent combined aortic and renal artery reconstruction as compared with a group of patients undergoing isolated aortic reconstruction. Note that fully 40% of patients who come to combined aortic/renal operation in contemporary practice have undergone some prior mechanical intervention for their coronary disease and such an aggressive posture towards the evaluation and treatment of associated coronary disease is an important factor in the cur-

Table 1.

Demographic and Clinical Features of 300 Patients Treated with Surgical Renal Artery Reconstruction.

Factor	%
Male sex	52
Age ≥ 70 years	29
Diabetes	14
Hypertension	95
Poorly controlled hypertension	51
Creatinine ≥ 1.5 mg/dL	53
Single functioning kidney	28
Coronary artery disease (evident clinically)	54

Table 2.

Evaluation and Management of Coronary Artery Disease in Patients Undergoing Aortic and Renovascular Surgery.

Variable	Combined Operation 1990–1994 (n = 60)		Isolated Aortic Surgery 1989–1990 (n = 202)		
	No.	%	No.	%	P Value
Patients with ≥ 2 CAD markers**	39	65	56	28	< 0.0001
% with preoperative D-Thal	35	58	58	29	< 0.0001
% with preoperative cor angio	17	28	16	8	< 0.0001
Preop PTCA/CABG	24	40	42	20	< 0.003

Combined operation = aortic graft with renal artery reconstruction; D-thal, Dipyridamole-thallium scintigraphy; cor angio, coronary angiography; PTCA, percutaneous coronary angioplasty. **CAD markers include diabetes, age of 70 years or older, and history of angina, myocardial infarction or congestive heart failure.

rent safety of surgical renal artery reconstruction. Accordingly, treatment decisions in patients with atherosclerotic RVD must consider not only the natural history of the renal artery lesion and its potential clinical sequelae but also the expected natural history of a patient typically afflicted with diffuse atherosclerosis.

Indications for Renal Artery Revascularization

In considering patients with atherosclerotic RVD, indications for treatment of renal artery stenosis (RAS) have shifted from primarily control of hypertension to revascularization for both hypertension control and salvage of renal function. Novick et al. documented more than a decade ago that the spectrum of indications for treatment of RVD had gradually shifted over the past 20 years. Whereas prior to 1985, fully half of renal artery reconstructions at the Cleveland Clinic were performed for hypertension control alone, in contemporary practice this figure had decreased to less than one-third of cases.[3] In a 1993 collective review, Rimmer detailed experience in some 500 patients treated for renal function salvage recording that 50% of patients treated had successful outcomes in terms of improvement in renal function, but another 20% either had deterioration in renal function or died as a complication of their treatment.[1] Parallel developments in the medical therapy of renovascular hypertension, while providing effective medical therapy for many patients, have also served to "unmask" patients with clinically occult, hemodynamically significant renal artery disease to the entire functioning renal mass. It is now recognized by most clinicians that the deterioration in renal excretory function after the introduction of ACE-inhibitor therapy is an important clinical clue to the presence of significant bilateral RAS.

The term ischemic nephropathy as originally defined by Dean et al. refers to the presence of renal excretory dysfunction in the presence of hemodynamically significant RAS.[4] Accordingly, this term defines a clinical circumstance rather than a pathologic entity. Patients with RVD typically have varying degrees of concomitant renal parenchymal pathology resulting from chronic hypertension, diabetic nephropathy in some, and chronic atheroembolism.[5] Such fixed and parenchymal pathology will often limit or indeed prevent benefit from renal revascularization. Imprecise patient stratification among important clinical, anatomic, and pathologic variables and failure to record clinically relevant endpoints and/or adequate follow-up have all contributed to confusion in the literature with respect to patients' inclusion and treatment results. While some authors have chosen some arbitrary level of renal dysfunction as the inclusion criteria,[6,7] we and others have considered revascularization to the entire functioning renal mass as an appropriate criteria to constitute revascularization for function salvage.[3,7,8]

The clinically important endpoints of patient survival and eventual dependence on dialysis can only be assessed from reports which contain adequate follow-up data. It is appropriate to emphasize at this point the extremely poor prognosis if atherosclerotic RVD progresses to end-stage renal failure (ESRD) and dialysis. Mailloux et al. in a series of important follow-up studies on ESRD patients indicated that those with RVD/atherosclerosis had a 50% mortality at just 2 years after initiation of dialysis therapy.[9] In our follow-up studies of 140 patients treated with surgical renal artery reconstruction for renal function salvage important features included the following: 1) clinical features especially those referable to renal dysfunction were, as expected, even more severe than those displayed in Table 1, i.e., a general population of patients undergoing renal revascularization. In patients treated for function salvage, 45% had a single functioning kidney, and 80% has some degree of renal insufficiency; 27% had extreme renal insufficiency (creatinine $\geq$ 3.0 mg/dL). Actuarial survival in patients treated for renal function salvage at 5 years was 52 $\pm$ 5%, significantly worse than a general cohort of patients treated for RVD (see Figure 1). Second, continued deterioration in renal function (despite anatomically successful renal artery repair) occurred in 24% of our patients with eventual dialysis in 15%. Survival after institution of dialysis was poor, with two-thirds of such patients deceased at follow-up. Continued deterioration of renal function was strongly correlated with increasing preoperative creatinine levels. The relative risk of continued deterioration of renal function was 1.6 (p = 0.001; 95% CI 1.2 to 1.8) for each 1.0 mg/dL increment in baseline creatinine levels. Stated differently and as displayed in Figure 2, continued deterioration in renal func-

$\longrightarrow$

Figure 2. Life-table analysis of likelihood of continued deterioration in renal function after anatomically successful renal artery repair performed for renal function salvage. A cohort of 140 patients was stratified according to baseline threshold creatinine of $\geq$ 3.0 mg/dL. Note the highly significant difference and the poor prognostic implications of baseline creatinine $\geq$ 3.0 mg/dL (reprinted with permission[24]).

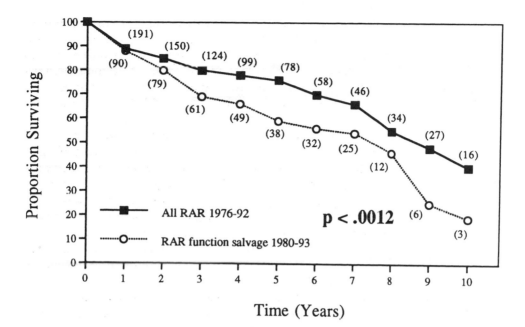

Figure 1. Comparative life-table survival curves for a series of 140 patients who underwent renal artery reconstruction (RAR) for renal function salvage, and a larger cohort of all patients undergoing surgical repair of atherosclerotic renovascular disease at the Massachusetts General Hospital over the interval 1976–1992. There is a significant (p < 0.0012) decrease in survival in those patients treated for renal function salvage (reprinted with permission[24]).

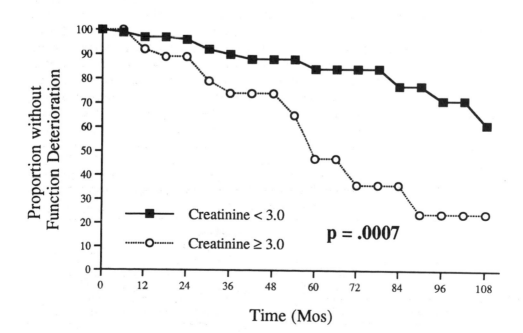

tion was striking (p = 0.0007) in those patients with extreme baseline renal insufficiency (creatinine ≥ 3.0 mg/dL). Other variables *inversely* associated with continued renal function deterioration were the notation of early postoperative improvement in renal function (≥ 20% decrement in creatinine) (RR=0.41; 95% CI 0.2–0.9, p = 0.04), and a significant reduction in postvascularization antihypertensive medication requirements (RR=0.03; 95% CI 0.0 to 0.5; p = 0.02).[8]

These sobering data emphasize the judgmental difficulties in the unsolved problem in RVD, namely predicting the functional response to revascularization. Despite the ominous implications of extreme (creatinine ≥ 3.0) baseline insufficiency, the dismal prognosis of those who come to dialysis and the overall favorable results in our patients (75% with improved/stable function over a mean 4 years follow-up) indicate that consideration of revascularization is appropriate. Dramatic results such as retrieval from dialysis dependence do occur; observational studies indicate further that rapid decline in renal function in the year prior to surgery, and comprehensive bilateral revascularization are findings suggestive of a favorable response to revascularization.[10,11] Clearly the general topic of which patients will benefit from revascularization is worthy of further prospective study, and those variables which should be considered in surgical decision making are listed in Table 3.

A commonly encountered clinical dilemma is the appropriate posture towards so-called "asymptomatic" or functionally silent RVD, which is discovered in the context of evaluation of vascular disease in other territories, and which may be accompanied by easily controlled hypertension.

Olin et al. emphasized that at least one-third of patients being evaluated for either aortic pathology or lower extremity occlusive disease with arteriography would be found to have greater than 50% stenosis in at least one renal artery and high grade bilateral disease was present in approximately 15% of patients.[12] Harding et al., reporting on a large series of patients undergoing coronary arteriography, and in whom abdominal aortograms were obtained at the conclusion of the procedure, noted that some degree of RAS was present in 30% of these patients and half of these had significant lesions. Similar to other reports, they found that the extent of coronary artery disease was related in linear fashion to the presence and severity of the RVD.[13] The clinical context of the patient's presentation has substantial bearing on the urgency and wisdom

---

Table 3.

Factors that Influence Success of Renal Revascularization for Function Salvage.

Clinical	*Anatomic*
Diabetes	Unilateral vs. bilateral revascularization
Comorbidities	Renal size
Rate of decline renal function	Status of renal parenchyma
Degree of baseline renal insufficiency	Intrarenal vascular changes
History atheroembolism syndrome	Stenotic vs. occluded vessel
Circumstances of clinical presentation	Vessel reconstitution beyond occlusion

---

of intervention for RVD. It is evident that many patients treated for RVD are at least initially referred for something other than clinical manifestations of RVD, in particular, aortic aneurysm or aortoiliac occlusive disease. There remains no consensus on the appropriate posture towards these patients. We and others have emphasized what could be considered an aggressive posture towards management of RVD in this setting (presuming the patient requires aortic surgery) with the fundamental argument for this approach referable to the favorable long term durability of a well performed surgical renal artery reconstruction when compared to the expected natural history of the disease untreated.[6,14,15] Alternatively, wholesale stenting of renovascular lesions detected during angiography is neither logical nor without the potential for complications.

The "conventional" wisdom dictates that intervention for RVD should only be undertaken when the RVD itself is functionally significant, irrespective of whether or not a coexistent aortic pathology mandates correction. Williamson et al. recently reported on a series of 200 patients who underwent aortic reconstruction and in whom so-called prophylactic renal artery reconstruction was avoided. Mean follow-up duration was 6.3 years. Fourteen percent of their patients had uncorrected high grade unilateral RAS and 5% had bilateral severe RAS. They noted at late follow-up that patients with RVD had increased hypertension and the need for antihypertensive medications, but no significant difference in survival rate, dialysis dependence or renal function deterioration when compared to those patients without RAS.[16] Interestingly, their survival rates for those with RAS (66%) were lower than those (84%) without RAS, but this difference did not achieve statistical significance. On the basis of this experience, the authors advised against prophylactic repair of RAS in patients undergoing aortic reconstruction. In the authors' opinion, this recommendation is overly conservative and the follow-up data in the Williamson study could have been anticipated since patients with any degree of renal insufficiency were excluded from the analysis.

At the extreme end of the wide spectrum of clinical presentations of RVD are those patients presenting with so-called "renovascular crises." We use this term to denote a variety of clinical presentations which include hypertensive crisis, hypertensive encephalopathy with or without lacunar infarction, rapidly progressive renal failure leading in some patients to the need for renal replacement therapy, and noncardiogenic pulmonary edema with severe hypertension and fluid overload. The latter patients are frequently discovered to have virtually normal cardiac *systolic* function and it is commonplace that these patients undergo an initial cardiac evaluation to rule out ischemic pulmonary edema and/or major impairment of left ventricular function. These patients typically have high grade RAS to the entire functioning renal mass and are in a state of avid sodium and fluid retention from secondary hyperaldosteronemia. Accordingly, the pulmonary edema typically responds well to loop diuretic therapy, but is often accompanied by a very narrow balance of intravascular volume, hypertension and renal excretory function. Overly aggressive diureses and/or lowering of the blood pressure tend to cause rapidly escalating azotemia. A dramatic clinical response to renal revascularization can be anticipated in this particular clinical scenario; in such circumstances we have often proceeded directly to surgical revascularization with magentic resonance angiography (MRA) as the sole preoperative imaging modality.[17,18]

Anatomy and Natural History of
Atherosclerotic Renovascular Disease

Certain factors referable to the anatomy of atherosclerotic RVD deserve emphasis. 1) 80% or more of RVD is so-called aortic "spillover" atherosclerosis, that is, an extension of aortic plaque that is at least partially ostial in nature and generally confined to the proximal 1–2 cm of the renal artery. 2) Aortic atherosclerosis, which is frequently underestimated by arteriography, often makes origination of aorto-renal bypass from the native aorta technically unsatisfactory. 3) RVD is frequently bilateral. In a review of nearly 300 patients treated at our institution, 50% or greater RAS occurred bilaterally in 40% of patients. However, only high-grade lesions, that is, greater than or equal to 75% diameter reduction will produce functionally significant alterations in renal blood flow. 4) Total proximal renal artery occlusion can occur with maintenance of renal viability via collateral circulation as seen on the late phase of arteriography or as inferred from the quality of the nephrogram obtained on a gadolinium enhanced MRA study.[18] In our series, 16% of repaired renal arteries had total proximal occlusion.[19]

Clinical decision making about the wisdom of intervention for atherosclerotic RVD, particularly in patients with functionally silent lesions or easily controlled hypertension, has traditionally been hampered by inadequate natural history data. Obviously, if a heretofore clinically quiescent renovascular lesion would remain so for the duration of the patient's lifetime, a conservative posture would seem appropriate. Judgments about the wisdom of proceeding with renovascular repair are predicated upon knowledge of the natural history of both the lesion and the patient without repair of the RAS. Most of the earlier natural history studies contain patients who were initially evaluated for hypertension with angiography, implying that these patients had at the point of entry functionally significant RVD. Only the recently reported study of Zierler et al, with sequential duplex scanning considered patients in prospective fashion.[20] The earlier angiographic studies were typically retrospective studies of patients who (either intentionally or not) had two angiographic studies available. Particularly germane to the clinical question of when to combine renal artery repair with aortic surgery is the study of Tollefson et al.[21] These investigators studied 27 patients who had two or more arteriograms performed at a mean interval of 4.5 years between studies with clinical follow-up that averaged 7 years. Despite the fact that the indications for patient entry were angiograms for aortic disease, the data with respect to lesion progression was at the upper range of that reported in the earlier studies. Most investigators have emphasized that arteries that proceeded to total occlusion harbored high grade stenoses at the time of initial evaluation and that progression to occlusion was not necessarily accompanied by deterioration in renal function. Obviously, this relates to the status of the contralateral kidney. The carefully conducted study of Schriber et al. emphasized that progression to occlusion was significantly correlated with high grade lesions at the time of initial study. Seventy percent of patients with lesions less than 50% stenosis showed no evidence of progression on follow-up study. This study did correlate lesion progression with evidence of clinical deterioration. In patients with lesion progression, over 50% had an increase in serum creatinine or increasing difficulty with blood pressure control.[22] Meaney et al. demonstrated that neither age, sex nor smoking history had any positive predictive value with respect to renal artery lesion progression.[23] Wollenwebber, et al. were the first to emphasize the overall cardiovascular risk associated with clinically significant RAS. They recorded an actuarial 5-year survival of 66% in their patients followed with RVD and emphasized that this was distinctly inferior to an age-matched normal patient population.[24] Our own data referable to patients who have undergone surgical renal artery repair indicated an actuarial survival of 75%, suggesting a favorable impact on life expectancy from treatment of RVD, but also identifying poor blood pressure control over time as a predictor of inferior long-term survival.[19] Only the study of Dean et al.[25] could be considered a randomized, prospective one in that they detailed the clinical course of 35 patients followed after initial randomization to medical therapy alone for angiographically documented renovascular hypertension. These investigators noted that 50% of their patients on medical therapy had deterioration of renal function irrespective of the ability of medical therapy to control blood pressure, a finding with particular significance in contemporary practice since the available medical armamentarium can frequently achieve reasonable blood pressure control in many patients with RVD.[25] The prospective duplex study of Zierler et al. detailed natural history data on 80 patients referred with either hypertension or renal insufficiency with a mean follow-up of 1 year. The cumulative incidence of progression from a less than to a greater than 60% RAS was 42% $\pm$ 14% at 2 years. For arteries initially noted to have greater than 60% stenosis, the rate of progression to total occlusion at two years was 11% $\pm$ 6% and disease progression was accompanied by poor control of diastolic blood pressure.[20]

Based on the available natural history information, the following conclusions are justified. First, lesion progression and accompanying clinical deterioration is common in patients with high grade (greater than 75% diameter reducing) atherosclerotic RVD. Second, following clinical parameters of blood pressure control and serum creatinine are unreliable predictors of the status of renal artery anatomy. Clinical deterioration frequently will represent progression to total renal artery occlusion at which point some irreversible loss of functioning renal parenchyma has likely already occurred.

Options for Surgical Renal
Artery Reconstruction

Surgical techniques for renal artery reconstruction have evolved as a function of anatomic and comorbidity considerations in patients with diffuse atherosclerosis. The contemporary vascular surgeon should be capable of applying the variety of reconstructions (as detailed in Table 4) in accordance with particular circumstances in individual patients. In addition to the anatomic

Table 4.

Options for Surgical Renal Artery Reconstruction.

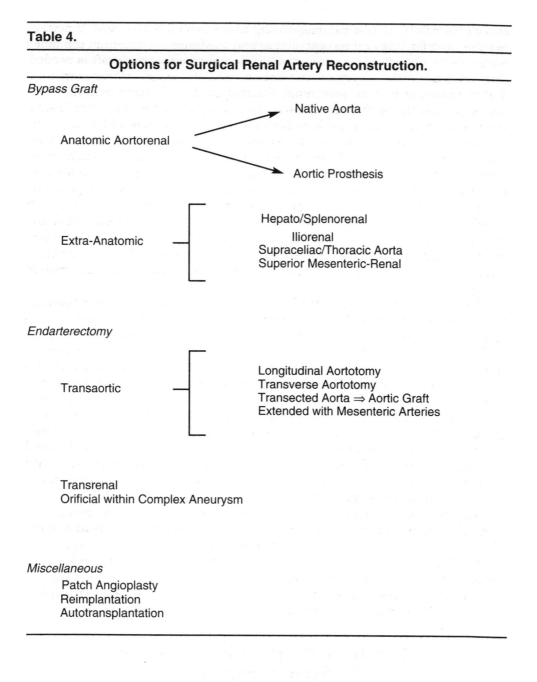

Bypass Graft

Anatomic Aortorenal
- Native Aorta
- Aortic Prosthesis

Extra-Anatomic
- Hepato/Splenorenal
- Iliorenal
- Supraceliac/Thoracic Aorta
- Superior Mesenteric-Renal

Endarterectomy

Transaortic
- Longitudinal Aortotomy
- Transverse Aortotomy
- Transected Aorta $\Rightarrow$ Aortic Graft
- Extended with Mesenteric Arteries

Transrenal
Orificial within Complex Aneurysm

Miscellaneous
  Patch Angioplasty
  Reimplantation
  Autotransplantation

factors referable to RVD as outlined above, the following clinical factors will influence the choice of renal artery reconstruction: 1) The degree of renal insufficiency. 2) The need for concomitant aortic replacement. 3) The need for contralateral nephrectomy. 4) The potential desirability of a staged approach in patients who require bilateral renal artery reconstruction. 5) Unilateral versus bilateral versus multiple renal arteries in need of reconstruction. 6) Age and

other comorbidity considerations. Among these variables, the most important
are the need for bilateral reconstruction and the issue of a potential combined
aortic and renal artery reconstruction. If an infrarenal aortic graft is needed,
then anatomic renal artery reconstruction either by means of transaortic endarterectomy, or with an aortorenal sidearm graft originating from the main
aortic graft, is the preferred technique. In the circumstance of bilateral reconstruction, we prefer transaortic endarterectomy, a technique which has experienced a "rebirth" in centers with considerable experience in renovascular
surgery. We noted a significant increase in the use of transaortic endarterectomy after 1990 especially in the circumstance of a bilateral repair, findings reported by others.[14,26] In the circumstance of unilateral renal artery repair combined with an infrarenal aortic graft, we prefer a sidearm aorto-renal graft
with end-to-end anastomosis to the renal artery. In contemporary practice,
combined aortic and renal artery grafting accounts for 50% of our renal artery
reconstructions. Follow-up studies have demonstrated that this an extremely
durable technique of reconstruction with a 5-year primary patency rate of
nearly 90%.[19]

Notable among trends in surgical renal artery reconstruction has been the
increased application of extra-anatomic reconstruction. While these reconstructions, particularly those based on the hepatic or splenic arteries, were initially applied in circumstances of considerable anatomic complexity such as
redo surgery, or when there was an absolute need to avoid surgical manipulation of the aorta, they have gradually evolved to a position of preferential use
in many patients when unilateral reconstruction is indicated. Our experience
has been that aorto-renal bypass originating from a heavily diseased native
aorta is both a considerable surgical undertaking, and has not performed well
in our hands. The overall surgical insult, in particular, with the hepato-renal
bypass on the right side, is considerably less than would be anticipated with
aorto-renal bypass. Accordingly, extra-anatomic reconstruction is particularly
well suited to high-risk patients.

Our perspective with the use of extra-anatomic reconstructions extends
some 25 years and in long term follow-up studies, we have demonstrated equivalent durability for these bypasses when compared to standard aorto-renal bypass.[19] Similar results have been reported from other centers of excellence.[27]
Indeed, the continuing preference for surgical renal artery reconstruction
when compared to endovascular revascularization is an argument principally
buoyed by the demonstrated durability of surgical reconstructions.

Results of Surgical Renal Artery Reconstruction

From an institutional perspective that extends nearly 25 years and involves nearly 500 renal artery reconstructions, certain principles have become
evident. Firstly, operative mortality, early graft failure, and the eventual need
for reoperation have been in the 5% range over this interval. In contemporary
practice, operative mortality is in the range anticipated for isolated elective
aortic surgical reconstruction (1%–2%). Interestingly, this figure is quite simi-

Table 5.

Contemporary Results of Surgical Renal Artery Reconstruction.

Author	Year	# Patients	% Combined Aortic Graft	Operative Mortality	Graft Patency
Hansen et al.[30]	1992	200	32	2.5	98%
Torsello et al.[31]	1990	326	50	4.3	94%
Cambria et al.[13]	1994	285	43	5.5	88% (5 yr)
Darling et al.[32]	1999	568	77	5.5	97%

lar to a recently reported large series of renal artery stenting.[28] Other contemporary clinical series which are notable for treatment of a preponderance of patients with atherosclerotic RVD detail similarly acceptable perioperative mortality rates in the 2%–5% range.[29–31] These data represent a substantial improvement over time in the overall risk of surgical renal artery reconstruction, and as displayed in Table 5, long-term patency has been most favorable. The majority of failures in renal artery reconstruction are technical in nature and occur in the early postoperative period. Therefore, a procedure tailored to individual patient anatomy and intended to avoid early technical problems is clearly an important factor in obtaining a durable result.

Favorable long-term anatomic results have been achieved with all types of renal artery reconstruction. Improvement in hypertension control has occurred in 80% of patients. It is uncommon to "cure" (i.e., normotensive, off of all medications) hypertension in patients with atherosclerotic RVD. Five-year actuarial survival after renal artery reconstruction has been greater than 70% in our patients, but the functional sequelae of RVD such as poorly controlled hypertension and advanced azotemia have been significant negative predictors of late survival.[19]

Angioplasty and Stent Placement for Renovascular Disease

Percutaneous renal artery angioplasty (PTA) was first described by Gruntzig in 1978.[32] The recent development of specialized diagnostic catheters, wires, balloon catheters, improved angiographic equipment, and metallic stents have facilitated many of the technical aspects of the procedure. Renal artery PTA has been applied with success to a spectrum of lesions ranging from fibromuscular dysplasia (FMD), atherosclerosis, and Takayasu's arteritis. The advent of metallic endovascular stents has fueled the drive towards more aggressive percutaneous management of RVD. In some centers, primary stenting of renal artery stenoses is the norm, rather than the exception.

Renal artery PTA should be performed to achieve specific clinical goals. The mere presence of a stenosis (with an angiographic catheter nearby), without consideration of the clinical status of the patient, is not an indication for percutaneous intervention. Clear definitions of the outcomes of angioplasty are essential to any discussion of the topic.[33] A technical success indicates a residual stenosis of less than 20%, hemodynamic improvement (diminished pressure gradient across the lesion), and no major morbidity. Clinical success refers to complete or substantial relief of the presenting symptom, be it hypertension, azotemia, or both. Patency rates describe the percentage of patients with technical and clinical success who remain symptomatically and angiographically improved.

Fibromuscular dysplasia, in particular the medial fibroplasia type, is perhaps the ideal lesion for percutaneous renal artery intervention for several reasons. Since FMD occurs in young, generally healthy individuals with otherwise normal arteries, the procedures are generally less complicated than would be in older patients with extensive atherosclerosis. In 1991, Tegtmeyer et al. reported a 100% technical success rate in 66 patients with 85 lesions treated with angioplasty for refractory renovascular hypertension.[34] The rate of cure (no further medications for hypertension) was 39%, with 59% improved and 2% with no response. Symptomatic restenosis occurred in 10%, however. The reported high technical and clinical success rates of angioplasty for FMD may explain the unsubstantiated impression that the majority of these lesions are treated by angioplasty in the community setting. Renal artery FMD has become a rare lesion in the vascular practice of most tertiary care referral centers.

The role of PTA in the management of atherosclerotic renal artery lesions has been controversial largely related to the anatomy (usually ostial) of atherosclerotic RVD. The current general enthusiasm for percutaneous vascular intervention now encompasses renal lesions as well. However, not all atherosclerotic renal artery lesions are the same, either in morphology or in response to percutaneous intervention. Atherosclerotic renal artery stenoses are classified by their location as either ostial or proximal lesions. Ostial renal artery stenoses are actually aortic wall plaque that encroaches upon the renal artery ostium. The conventional definition is that any lesion within 1 cm of the aortic lumen should be considered ostial. Proximal renal artery stenoses involve the main renal artery at least 1 cm beyond the ostium. The location of proximal atherosclerotic plaque is within the renal artery proper. This classification is useful when contemplating renal artery interventions, but in practice distinction between types may be difficult, and both lesions may be present simultaneously.

Proximal renal artery atherosclerotic stenoses respond very well to angioplasty, although not as well as FMD. Most series report an 80% technical success rate, with a 68%–90% clinical success rate, and 5-year patency rates as high as 88%.[35] In the only prospective randomized comparison of renal artery PTA with surgery, the 2-year primary patency after angioplasty was 75%, but increased to 90% after secondary interventions.[36] Patients with atherosclerotic lesions undergoing renal artery angioplasty for hypertension have a lower rate of cure than FMD, although fully 50% experience better blood pressure control.[35,36] A 20% reduction in pretreatment creatinine in patients with renovascular azotemia can be achieved in approximately half of patients after PTA of bilateral RAS or stenosis in the artery to a single kidney.[37] Angioplasty of unilateral RAS in patients with two kidneys and azotemia provides no benefit in stabilization of renal dysfunction.

Angioplasty of ostial atherosclerotic stenoses has a low rate of technical success (10%–35%), due to the elastic nature of the aortic wall plaque. Although one study suggested that almost 60% of patients experienced clinical benefit despite suboptimal technical results,[35] most interventionalists have a low expectation for success with angioplasty alone in ostial lesions. Of interest is a recent report from the Emory group focusing on renal PTA with stent placement in 73 patients. While technical success (including secondary procedures at the initial procedures) was high at 94%, major complications occurred in 97% and restenosis at 1 year occurred in 16%.[38]

Overall reported complication rates of renal artery PTA in contemporary series are generally low but will be strongly influenced by patient selection.[39] Rates at specific institutions will be different depending on the case mix and operator skill. It is important to note that the literature on angioplasty alone of atherosclerotic renal artery stenoses becomes somewhat thin after 1990 due to the advent of metallic stents.

Metallic stents are now widely used in the treatment of renal artery stenoses. Although the dispassionate observer would argue that their exact role remains to be defined, stents are now synonymous with percutaneous renal artery intervention. The driving force behind the liberal use of stents is the high technical success that can be achieved when stents are applied to salvage failed angioplasty.[40] The natural (but not necessarily correct) assumption is that the use of stents in all patients (i.e., "primary stenting") would therefore improve the overall outcomes of angioplasty. Dorros et al. reported a 25% restenosis rate in a series of 76 patients who underwent primary renal artery stenting for mixed indications.[41] The results of a more conservative approach were reported by Blum et al. in 1997 in a series of 68 patients treated for renovascular hypertension.[42] Stents were used for ostial renal artery lesions only after angioplasty failed to meet hemodynamic and angiographic criterion for success. This group reported a 100% technical success rate, with an 84% primary patency at 60 months, and a 92% secondary patency, and a restenosis rate of 11%. These results were achieved with a remarkably low complication rate (three hematomas, but no episodes of postprocedural renal failure). The high technical success was remarkable in that these patients would have otherwise been considered angioplasty failures. Clinical benefit was realized in 78% of the patients. Similarly encouraging results with renal artery stents have been reported in patients with azotemia and RAS as the chief indication for intervention;[43] however, the balance of contemporary reports—particularly those from centers of excellence, reveal a consistent theme of failing to demonstrate improvement in excretory function after percutaneous revascularization.[28,38,42] It is the author's opinion that such circumstances represent judgmental rather than technical failures.

Surgery Versus Angioplasty at the Millennium

It is our opinion that a review of the available data, and with the perspective of extensive experience in managing atherosclerotic RVD the following conclusions are justified. Firstly, there is no "level one" evidence (i.e., prospective randomized trials) indicating the superiority of surgical versus endovascular renal revascularization. Second, the availability of stenting has vastly improved the unfavorable results of PTA alone for renal ostial lesions. Despite this consideration, surgical revascularization remains the standard with respect to durability considerations. Third, procedural morbidity and mortality, while intuitively expected to favor percutaneous revascularization, is quite variable in the extant literature, peri-procedural mortality in certain large series of stenting, is in the range anticipated for surgery in contemporary practice.[28]

It is out posture that both surgical revascularization and stenting are valid and effective techniques for renal revascularization. Similar to judgments in other vascular territories, the mode of intervention is selected after a comprehensive consideration of individual patient age, anatomy, clinical circumstance and co-morbidity. Thorough understanding and sophistication in these spheres is a requirement for those who profess technical ability to treat atherosclerotic RVD.

References

1. Rimmer JM, Grennari FJ. Atherosclerotic renovascular disease and progressive renal failure. *Annals Intern Med* 1993; 118:712–719.
2. Valentine RJ, Clagett GP, Miller GL, et al. The coronary risk of unsuspected renal artery stenosis. *J Vasc Surg* 1993; 18:433–440.
3. Novick AC, Ziegelbaum M, Vidt DG, et al. Trends in surgical revascularization for renal artery disease. Ten year's experience. *JAMA* 1987; 257:498–501.
4. Dean RH, Englund R, Dupont WD, et al. Retrieval of renal function by revascularization. Ann Surg 1985; 202:367–374.
5. Vidt DG, Eisele G, Gephardt GN, et al. Atheroembolic renal disease: Association with renal artery stenosis. *Cleve Clinic J Med* 1989; 56(4): 407–413.
6. Chaikof EL, Smith RB, Salam AA, et al. Ischemic neuropathy and concomitant aortic disease: a 10-year study. *J Vasc Surg* 1994; 19:135–148.
7. Libertino JA, Bosco PJ, Ying Cy, et al. Renal revascularization to preserve and restore renal function. *J Urol* 1992; 147:1485–1487.
8. Cambria RP, Brewster DC, L'Italien G, et. al. Renal artery reconstruction for the preservation of renal function. *J Vasc Surg* 1996: 24: 371–382.
9. Mailloux LU, Bellucci AG, Mossey RT, et al. Predictors of survival in patients undergoing dialysis. *Am J Med* 1988; 84:855–862.
10. Hansen KJ, Thomason RB, Craven TE, et al. Surgical management of dialysis-dependent ischemic nephropathy. *J Vasc Surg* 1995; 21:197–211.
11. Dean RH, Tribble RW, Hansen KJ, et al. Evolution of renal insufficiency in ischemic nephropathy. *Ann Surg* 1991; 2:13:446–455.
12. Olin JM, Melia M, Young JR, et al. Prevalence of atherosclerotic renal artery stenosis in patients with atherosclerosis elsewhere. *Am J Med* 1990; 88:46–51.
13. Harding MD, Smith LR, Himmelstein SI, et al. Renal artery stenosis: Prevalence and associated risk factors in patients undergoing routine cardiac catheterization. *J Am Soc Neph* 1992; 2:1608–1616.
14. Cambria RP, Brewster DC, L'Italien G, et al. Simultaneous aortic and renal artery reconstruction: Evolution of an eighteen-year experience. *J Vasc Surg* 1995; 21:916–925.
15. Allen BT, Rubin BG, Anderson CB, et al. The simultaneous surgical management of aortic and renovascular disease. *Am J Surg* 1993; 166:726–733.

16. Williamson WK, Abou-Zamzam Jr. AM, Moneta GL, et al. Prophylactic repair of renal artery stenosis is not justified in patients who require infrarenal aortic reconstruction. *J Vasc Surg* 1998; 28:14–22.

17. Riemont MJ, Kaufman JA, Geller SC, et. al. Evaluation of renal artery stenosis with dynamic gadolinium-enhanced magnetic resonance angiography. *Am J Radiol* 1997; 169:39–44.

18. Cambria RP, Kaufman JA, Brewster DC, et al. Surgical renal artery reconstruction without angiography; the role of clinical profiling and magnetic resonance angiography. *J Vasc Surg* 1999; 29(6):1012–1021.

19. Cambria RP, Brewster DC, L'Italien GJ, et al. The durability of different reconstructive techniques for atherosclerotic renal artery disease. *J Vasc Surg* 1994; 20:76–87.

20. Zierler RE, Bergelin RO, Isaacson JA, et al. Natural history of atherosclerotic renal artery stenosis: A prospective study with duplex ultrasound. *J Vasc Surg* 1994; 19:250–258.

21. Tollefson DF, Ernst CB. Natural history of atherosclerotic renal artery stenosis associated with aortic disease. *J Vasc Surg* 1991; 14:327–331.

22. Schreiber MJ, Pohl MA, Novick AC. The natural history of atherosclerotic and fibrous renal artery disease. *Urol Clin North Am* 1984; 11:383–392.

23. Meaney TF, Dustan HP, McCormack LJ. Natural history of renal artery disease. *Radiology* 1968; 91:881–887.

24. Wollenweber J, Sheps SG, Davis GD. Clinical course of atherosclerotic renovascular disease. *Am J Cardiol* 1968; 21:60–71.

25. Dean RH, Kieffer RW, Smith BM, et al. Renovascular hypertension: Anatomic and renal function changes during drug therapy. *Arch Surg* 1981; 116:1408–1415.

26. Hallett JW Jr, Textor SC, Kos PB, et al. Advanced renovascular hypertension and renal insufficiency: Trends in medical comorbidity and surgical approach from 1970 to 1993. *J Vasc Surg* 1995; 21:750–760.

27. Reilly JM, Rubin BG, Thompson RW, et al. Long term effectiveness of extra-anatomic renal artery revascularization. *Surgery* 1994; 116:784–791.

28. Rodriuez-Lopez JA, Werner A, Ray LI, et al. Renal artery stenosis treated with stent deployment: Indications, technique and outcome for 108 patients. *J Vasc Surg* 1999; 29:617–624.

29. Hansen KJ, Star SM, Sands RE, et al. Contemporary surgical management of renovascular disease. *J Vasc Surg* 1992; 16:319–331.

30. Torsello G, Sachs M, Kniemeyer H, et al. Results of surgical treatment for atherosclerotic renovascular occlusive disease. *Eur J Vasc Surg* 1990; 4:477–482.

31. Darling RC, Krerenberg PB, Chang BB, et al. Outcome of renal artery reconstruction: an analysis of 687 procedures. *Ann Surg* (in press).

32. Gruntzig A, Kuhlmann U, Vetter W, et al. Treatment of renovascular hypertension with percutaneous transluminal dilatation of a renal-artery stenosis. *Lancet* 1978; 1:801–802.

33. Standards of Practice Committee of the Society of Cardiovascular and Interventional Radiology. Guidelines for percutaneous transluminal angioplasty. *Radiology* 1990; 177:619–626.

34. Tegtmeyer CJ, Selby JB, Hartwell GD, et al. Results and complications of angioplasty in fibromuscular disease. *Circulation* 1991; 83(2 Suppl): 155–161.

35. Martin LG, Cork RD, Kaufman SL. Long-term results of angioplasty in 110 patients with renal artery stenosis. *JVIR* 1992; 3; 619–626.

36. Weibull H, Berqvist D, Bergentz S-E, et al. Percutaneous transluminal angioplasty versus surgical reconstruction of atherosclerotic renal artery stenosis: A prospective randomized study. *J Vasc Surg* 1993; 18:841–852.

37. Losimo F, Zuccala A, Busato F, et al. Renal artery angioplasty for renovascular hypertension and preservation of renal function: Long-term angiographic and clinical follow-up. *AJR* 1994; 162:853–857.

38. Bush RL, MacDonald MJ, Lin PH, et al. Endovascular revascularization of renal artery stenosis: Technical and clinical results. Presented at the 24ᵗʰ annual meet-

ing of the Southern Association for Vascular Surgery, Tucson, Arizona Jan 19–22, 2000.

39. Libertino JA, Beckmann CF. Surgery and percutaneous angioplasty in the management of renovascular hypertension. *Urologic Clin N Amer* 1994; 21:235–243.
40. Rees CR, Palmaz JC, Becker GJ, et al. Palmaz stent in atherosclerotic stenoses involving the ostia of the renal arteries: Preliminary report of a multicenter study. *Radiology* 1991; 181:507–514.
41. Dorros G, Jaff M, Jain A, et al. Follow-up of primary Palmaz-Schatz stent placement for atherosclerotic renal artery stenosis. *Am J Card* 1995; 75:1051–1055.
42. Blum U, Krumme B, Flugel P, et al. Treatment of ostial renal artery stenoses with vascular endoprostheses after unsuccessful balloon angioplasty. *N Engl J Med* 1997; 336:459–465.
43. Rundback JH, Gray RJ, Rozenblit G, et al. Renal artery stent placement for the management of ischemic nephropathy. *J Vasc Interv Radiol* 1998; 9:413–420.

9

Can Renal Artery Stenting Preserve Renal Function?

An Analysis of the Present Data, and Issues for Future Investigation

Stephen C. Textor, MD and Michael McKusick, MD

Introduction

Atherosclerotic renal artery stenosis (RAS) as a potential cause of renal failure continues to present major challenges to clinicians caring for patients with cardiovascular disease. Particularly since the wide introduction of potent antihypertensive agents, such as angiotensin converting enzyme inhibitors, angiotensin receptor blockers and calcium channel blockers, resistant hypertension alone is less commonly the pressing indication for renal revascularization than before.[1] In its place has come the concern that progressive vascular occlusive disease may threaten the viability of the post-stenotic kidney, placing the patient at risk for irreversible loss of renal function. Such renal damage due to underperfusion of the kidneys has been designated "ischemic nephropathy."

Central to the perception that ischemic nephropathy is indeed related to the vascular lesion is the potential to arrest or reverse this process by restoring renal blood flow. Clinical observations of recovery of renal function after successful renal revascularization, either by surgical or endovascular methods, has lent credence to this paradigm.[2] The introduction and application of stents to atherosclerotic lesions, particularly those near the renal ostia, offer the po-

From Jaff MR (ed): *Endovascular Therapy for Atherosclerotic Renal Artery Stenosis: Present and Future*. Armonk, NY: Future Publishing Co, Inc.; ©2001.

tential to widen the population in whom restoration of renal blood flow is possible.[3]

This chapter will undertake to provide an overview of the epidemiologic and clinical data supporting these concerns. It will seek further to identify data regarding the progression of renovascular disease in the current era and to examine the potential role for invasive endovascular procedures to improve renal function. It should be emphasized that precise rates of disease progression and precise estimates of benefits of intervention remain in flux with the introduction of ever more sophisticated therapy. As a result, experienced clinicians may disagree as to the relative merits of each approach. Where such disagreements prevail, we will seek to identify the key areas in which further data are needed.

Vascular Occlusive Disease as a Threat to Renal Function

Occluded renal arteries have been known for years to be associated with renal atrophy and scarring. Early reports of vascular repair after acute renal artery obstruction emphasized that renal function could be restored, if revascularization could be achieved soon enough.[4] In recent years, vascular compromise related to high-grade stenotic lesions have been observed to produce loss of renal size,[5] reduce blood flow, and to induce parenchymal fibrogenic responses. The mechanisms underlying renal damage in this setting are not yet clear. Most experimental and clinical studies indicate that such changes develop at levels of "critical perfusion" pressures at which point hemodynamic changes beyond the stenotic kidney do indeed reduce perfusion pressures and usually blood flow.[6] However, the kidney is supplied with a vast excess of oxygenated blood relative to its metabolic needs. In this respect, it differs considerably from either the brain or heart. Measurements of oxygen tension and erythropoetin levels in such hypoperfused kidneys do not support an overall deprivation of oxygen.[7] Localized areas of true "ischemia" within the kidney cannot be excluded but have been rarely observed. The mechanisms by which reduced arterial perfusion, despite adequate overall oxygenation, leads to kidney tissue fibrosis remain to be fully defined and represent a major gap in our understanding of this disease.

Patients with high-grade renal artery stenotic lesions to both kidneys or to a solitary functioning kidney may develop progressive renal failure. We have observed some patients who progressed to end-stage renal failure (ESRD) with no other identified renal disease.[6,8] Such patients are considered to have "ischemic nephropathy" primarily and have been the subject of considerable attention in recent years.[9,10] Remarkably, patients above age 50 years with other manifestations of vascular disease and no other identifiable renal diagnosis may comprise between 8%–15% of new Caucasian patients reaching ESRD in the United Kingdom and the United States.[11] The incident rate of patients needing renal replacement therapy has been increasing in recent years, most strikingly in patients in older age groups, often with diabetes and other manifestations of large vessel atherosclerosis. Such observations have stimulated some authors to recommend "screening" and to consider renal revascularization on a routine basis in newly identified patients with advanced renal dysfunction.

Incidental Renal Arterial Stenosis

Recent studies in patients undergoing coronary angiography or peripheral arterial angiography re-emphasize the generalized nature of atherosclerosis. Patients with widespread atherosclerotic disease involving the lower extremities or aorta, tend to have identifiable RAS in 40%–50% of cases.[12] Some degree of RAS is present in 30% of patients with coronary disease. Because such lesions are detected "incidentally" as part of a vascular study for other reasons, we designate these "incidental RAS." How often such lesions represent an important causative factor related to either hypertension and/or other cardiovascular morbidity is controversial. Follow-up studies in large cohorts with RAS identified during coronary angiography suggest that the presence of renovascular disease indeed predicts increased mortality during 4 years of follow-up.[13] Mortality in such cases is related primarily to cardiovascular events including stroke, myocardial infarction and congestive heart failure. However, the incidence of progressive renal dysfunction in this cohort is negligible.

Progression of Renal Artery Stenosis

Fundamental to the discussion of ischemic nephropathy is the tendency of vascular occlusion from atherosclerosis to become more severe with time. Factors governing the rates of progression are not well understood, although risk factors related to diabetes, level of blood pressure control and cholesterol homeostasis are likely to be important in the renal vasculature, as elsewhere.[14,15] How often such lesions progress to "critical" levels is also controversial, and may indeed be changing. Retrospective series from studies of serial aortographic studies obtained during the 1970s and 1980s suggest rates of 40%–50% progression in important "steps" over 4–5 year intervals.[16,17] Total occlusion of the renal artery was 15%–16% in these series. Prospective studies obtained with cohorts identified in the early 1990s, however, demonstrate lower overall rates of progression approximately 20%–25% overall during 2.5–3 years of follow-up. Progression to total occlusion was 7% in these series.[18]

Progression of clinical renal insufficiency also has been infrequent. Recent prospective studies of patients treated either with medical regimens or renal revascularization have encountered progressive renal failure rarely.[19,20]

Undeniably, some patients do develop progressive renovascular disease, which must be recognized as a group of discernible "renovascular syndromes." Such patients present with features of deteriorating blood pressure control, rising levels of serum creatinine (occasionally manifest as acute renal insufficiency during antihypertensive therapy) and/or episodes of rapidly developing circulatory congestion ("flash" pulmonary edema). These features often represent extension of renovascular disease to both kidneys and/or dependence on a solitary functioning kidney.

Revascularization to Restore Renal Function

Trends in both surgical and endovascular intervention in the renal arteries have shifted toward patients with progressive renal dysfunction over the past decade.[21,22] More than 50% of patients have such an indication in many centers. Surgical revascularization in our institution included approximately 30% of patients with serum Creatinine levels above 2.0 mg/dL in the period between 1980 and 1993.[21] Recent reports from series of stent application reflect similar figures.

Restoration of patency to renal vessels can indeed allow improvement in renal function. This can be achieved either with surgery,[23] percutaneous transluminal renal angioplasty (PTRA) alone,[24] or PTRA with application of stents.[25] An example of improved renal function after stenting a patient with a solitary functioning kidney is illustrated in Figure 1. When this occurs, improvement in renal function can be durable for many years. As noted in our series of patients with improved renal function, serum creatinine fell from 4.8 ± 0.6 mg/dL to 2.4 ± 0.3 mg/dL during a follow-up period of 27 months.[1] Relief of the stenosis removes the concern about post-stenotic renal atrophy during further antihypertensive therapy and may allow the safe use of angiotensin converting enzyme inhibitors, for example, in patients with congestive cardiac failure.[26] Occasional reports emphasize the potential for **proteinuria** to develop in patients with renal artery stenosis.[27] When proteinuria exceeds three grams daily, the rate of progressive renal failure accelerates and becomes more clearly dependent upon arterial pressures, regardless of the underlying renal disease. Recent trials of ACE inhibitors and other antihypertensive agents in patients with chronic renal disease demonstrate that reduction of proteinuria is an important predictor in slowing the rate of renal disease progression.[28] Remarkably, occasional reports of heavy proteinuria associated with renal artery stenosis demonstrate reversal of proteinuria after successful revascularization or nephrectomy.[27,29] Although this is an indirect observation, it reinforces the concept that restoration of renal perfusion under these circumstances provides an important mechanism for protecting the kidney.

How often and how consistently does renal function improve after restoring patency of the renal artery? Changes in renal function after any of these procedures have been difficult to evaluate in any simple fashion. On average, serum creatinine and where measured, glomerular filtration rates, remain "unchanged" for the majority of patients. Table 1 summarizes seven published series with a total of 556 patients treated with endovascular stents.[25,26,30–34] The precise figures regarding renal function vary depending upon criteria used to identify "changes" in creatinine (often presented as a change in creatinine in either relative or absolute terms, ranging from as little as 0.2 mg/dL to 1.0 mg/dL). In all of these reports, group mean creatinine values do not change during follow-up periods ranging from 6 months to several years. Our own analysis of 253 patients undergoing PTRA for atheroscle-

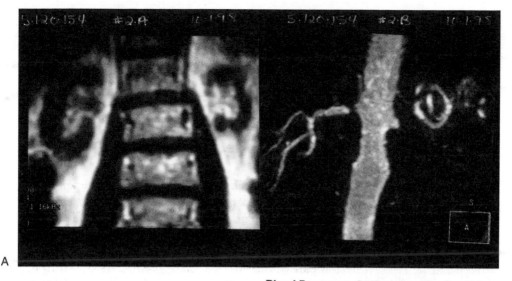

A

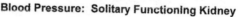

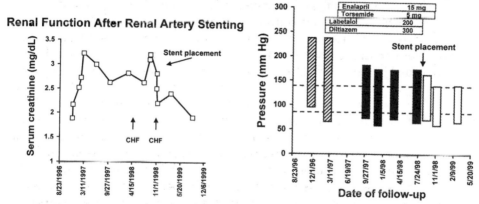

B

Figure 1. Blood pressure levels and kidney function in a patient with solitary functioning kidney managed both with medical therapy and after stent placement: (a) Magnetic resonance angiogram demonstrating total occlusion of the left renal artery and a high-grade occlusion to the right kidney in an 87-year-old man with deteriorating kidney function. (b) Blood pressure levels and progression of renal dysfunction during medical therapy in the same patient. He wished to avoid interventional procedures and was managed for 2 years with medical therapy alone. Blood pressure (left panel) control was possible with high doses of multiple antihypertensive medications, although it was associated with a rise in creatinine to 3.3 mg/dL. Development of multiple episodes of circulatory congestion ("flash" pulmonary edema labeled as "CHF" in the right panel) led to placement of an endovascular stent to restore blood flow to the solitary right kidney. Kidney function has improved as shown by a fall in creatinine to 1.9 mg/dL, blood pressure is more easily treated and he has had no further episodes of pulmonary vascular congestion.

Table 1.

Summary of Changes in Kidney Function after Percutaneous Renal Stent Placement in Atherosclerotic Renal Artery Stenosis.

Author	No. Pts.	F/U	Age	Creatinine Pre	Creatinine Post	Criteria	Reste-nosis	Improved	Stable	Worse	Diabetes	
Dorros 1998	145	>6 mos 4 years	67	2	1.8	>0.2 mg/dL	Bilateral	33 35	33 29	34 35	27%	Note: 38% >1.5 mg/dL 99% technological success >2.0 mg/dL: 3.6% bilateral 33% unilateral Note: ? restenosis rate Rel poor survival/5 years
Gross 1998	30	>6 mos	65.5	1.47	1.39	>0.2 mg/dL	12.50%	9/29 (31%)	15/29 (51.70%)	12/30 (40%)		
Blum 1997	68	27 mos	60	1.23	"No change"	10%					4/68 (5.80%)	Bilat = 6
White 1997	100		67 Total	Azotemic: 2.4 1.8	2.5 1.8	Bilat = 33 Unilat = 67	22.50%					Indications: CRF = 44% 99% technical success Clinical success = 76%
Tuttle 1998	129	24 mos	71	40 (GFR) Subgroups 53 26	39 43 23		14%					4/8 left dialysis dependence Bilat = 15% Unilat = 78% Sol. kidney = 7%
Runback 1998	45	17 mos	70	2.10	2.05*	20%	N/A	20%	52	28%	31%	All patients ≥ 1.5 mg/dL
Xue 1999	39	12 mos	68	1.71	1.53			10%	71%	8%		None left dialysis
Total	556											

*presented only for those with "benefit". In none of these series was an overall improvement change in kidney function noted. F/U = follow-up.

rosis, of which 44 had renal dysfunction (creatinine >2.0 mg/dL), is consistent with these reports and many others in the literature: On average, serum creatinine does not change, despite technically successful renal artery reconstruction (Figure 2A).

Average values for the group are misleading, however. These fail to identify important clinical benefits in patients whose renal function improves from advanced renal failure needing dialytic support which return to near normal levels. These patients are illustrated in the left panel of Figure 2B, in which creatinine fell from 4.8 ± 0.6 mg/dL to 2.3 ± 0.3 mg/dL. At least one series of patients with endovascular stent intervention reported four of eight patients removed from dialysis after restoring renal blood flow.[25] It must be emphasized that such patients are a minority, however, ranging from 25%–30% in most series. Nearly 50% of patients subjected to revascularization will have no meaningful change in kidney function during long-term follow-up, as illustrated in the middle panel of Figure 2B. Various authors interpret these patients in various ways. Commonly, they are considered to have "stabilized" renal function, implicitly because they no longer face the hazard of progressive vascular oc-

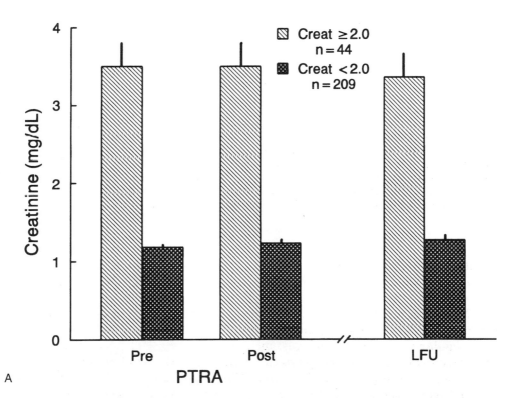

Figure 2. (a) Serum creatinine levels in n = 253 subjects with atherosclerotic renal artery stenosis before (pre), immediately after (post) and at last follow-up (LFU, mean 25 mos.) after technically successful PTRA. The left-hand bars represent 44 azotemic patients (defined as serum creatinine ≥ 2.0 mg/dL). Mean levels of creatinine did not change for the group either immediately after the procedure or during long-term follow-up. (*continued*)

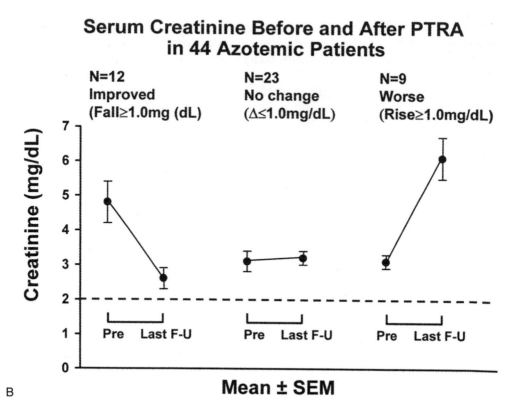

Figure 2. (*continued*) (b) Subgroups from the group of 44 azotemic subjects: Clinical improvement was defined as a reduction in serum creatinine ≥ 1.0 mg/dL, whereas "worse" was defined as a rise in creatinine by the same amount. As with most series of both surgical and endovascular renal artery intervention, group mean values do not change because distinct clinical subgroups offset each other. Despite a major improvement in 12 subjects, mean values were unchanged because of deteriorating renal function in 9/44 (20.5%). The largest group had no major change in renal function and is usually considered to have "stabilized" renal function.

clusion which might have occurred had they not been treated. Whether they truly face such hazard and how much they gain is controversial, as noted above.

Most problematic, however, is the group of patients whose renal function deteriorates substantially during the period after revascularization. This occurs regularly with all procedures, including surgery, PTRA and the use of stents (see Table 1). This group typically is between 18%–25% of subjects. It is the presence of this group which prevents the inference of an overall group benefit and leaves the mean level of creatinine "unchanged." These patients are presented variously as "failures," or "no benefit" or "worse." It is remarkable how constant the size of this group remains, regardless of the specific method of renal revascularization used. It is likely that technical failure alone cannot account for these events. Undoubtedly some of these patients lose kidney function from localized atheroembolic complications. Other mechanisms, as yet undefined, related to abrupt restoration of blood flow may contribute to renal functional deterioration also. As a result, the clinician must consider that renal revascularization offers a small but genuine risk of accelerating renal deterioration.

Some reports suggest that the rate of decline of renal function (expressed as reciprocal creatinine plots over time), rather than glomerular filtration alone, is slowed by successful stent placement.[35] The few prospective, randomized studies available regarding renal revascularization have not yet confirmed this premise.[19,20,36]

Prediction of the results of renal revascularization in a specific patient remains an elusive goal. Numerous reports indicate that "small" kidneys as determined by radiographic or ultrasound imaging are less likely to recover function than larger kidneys. Most series emphasize that advanced levels of renal dysfunction, as reflected by serum creatinines above 3.0 mg/dL predict less favorable responses.[21] The presence of older age, gradual loss of kidney function, widespread atherosclerotic disease of the aorta, and diabetes all predict less favorable outcome. There are, however, exceptions to all of these observations. Occasional reports appear of patients with advanced renal failure receiving dialysis therapy who recover sufficient function to be removed from dialysis.[37] Some authors observe that those patients with more recent loss of renal function, for example those with a rise of serum creatinine within a few months prior to revascularization, are more likely to recover function than those with slow, progressive loss of function.[38] Others note that collateral circulation may play an important role, as evidenced by reconstitution of blood flow beyond an occluded or stenotic lesion or the presence of a nephrogram on imaging studies.

There are no specific studies to assure a favorable outcome within the kidney. An important area of research is to examine the factors by which underperfusion of the kidney becomes a stimulus to progressive fibrogenesis.[39] Initial data from experimental studies indicate that vascular stenosis can alter levels of oxidative stress within the kidney, which is known to fuel activation of inflammatory cytokines and promotors of scarring in other renal diseases. Whether these will provide practical guidelines to identifying kidneys both (1) at risk for progressive parenchymal injury and (2) likely to benefit from restoration of blood flow are important questions yet to be answered.

Can Renal Artery Stents Preserve Renal Function?

The issues discussed above apply generally to the problem of critical renal artery stenosis from atherosclerosis. Clinical data until now indicate that restoration of renal perfusion by any means, whether using endovascular stents or surgical revascularization offer the same potential benefits during the short term. Both carry some risks. There are as yet no prospective comparisons between stenting and surgical intervention related to renal function. Proponents of surgical revascularization present long-term follow-up data regarding the "durability" of renal vessels remaining patent over many years.[40,41] Although the initial risks and costs of stenting are lower than surgery, restenosis due to intimal hyperplasia and development of stenosis at a site of vascular motion are recognized limitations. These occur at rates ranging between 12%–40% or more within the first year, depending upon local experience and other factors. Often these can be addressed with further endovascular procedures.

Reports of results regarding changes in renal function in current series using endovascular stents are limited to relatively short time. Whether long-term results will make them attractive alternatives to surgery in patients with otherwise long life expectancies remains to be determined.

Future Investigation Regarding Endovascular Stents and Renal Function

Taken together, the introduction of endovascular stents for the renal artery represents a major step forward to offering percutaneous intervention to patients with atherosclerosis. A major limitation in older patients had been the ostial location of this disease and its tendency to recoil after simple angioplasty. Many of these patients have comorbid diseases with enough added cardiovascular risk to render reconstructive surgery impractical. As both expertise and stent design advance, these tools will be applied more freely to patients developing progressive renal artery stenosis. The central technical issues will concern how to minimize vessel restenosis and trauma, while restoring adequate renal perfusion. Critical areas for research will focus on patient selection and identification of patients both at risk for progressive renal injury and likely to improve with restoration of vessel patency.

References

1. Textor SC. Revascularization in atherosclerotic renal artery disease. *Kidney Int* 1998; 53:799–811.
2. Novick AC. Patient selection for intervention to preserve renal function in ischemic renal disease. In Novick AC, Scoble J, Hamilton G (eds): **Renal Vascular Disease**. London: W.B.Saunders Co.,LTD., 1996, pp 323–337.
3. Palmaz JC. The current status of vascular intervention in ischemic nephropathy. *J Vasc Intervent Radiology* 1998; 9:539–543.
4. Vulcan T, Wilson M, Johnston W, et al. Restoration of renal function by arterial surgery. *Lancet* 1974; 1:653–656.
5. Caps MT, Zierler RE, Polissar NL, et al. Risk of atrophy in kidneys with atherosclerotic renal artery stenosis. *Kidney Int* 1998; 53:735–742.
6. Textor SC, Novick A, Tarazi RC, et al. Critical perfusion pressure for renal function in patients with bilateral atherosclerotic renal vascular disease. *Ann Int Med* 1985; 102:309–314.
7. Textor SC, Smith-Powell L. Pathophysiology of renal failure in ischemic renal disease. In Novick AC, Scoble J, Hamilton G (eds): **Renal Vascular Disease**. London: W.B. Saunders, 1996, pp 289–302.
8. Scoble JE, Maher ER, Hamilton G, et al. Atherosclerotic renovascular disease causing renal impairment- A case for treatment. *Clinical Nephrology* 1989; 31:119–122.
9. Mailloux LU, Napolitano B, Bellucci AG, et al. Renal vascular disease causing end-

stage renal disease: Incidence, clinical correlates, and outcomes: A 20-year clinical experience. *Am J Kidney Dis* 1994; 24:622–629.

10. Breyer JA, Jacobson HR. Ischemic Nephropathy. *Curr Opin Nephrol Hyper* 1993; 2:216–224.
11. Connolly JO, Higgins RM, Walters HL, et al. Presentation, clinical features and outcome in different patterns of atherosclerotic renovascular disease. *Q J Med* 1994; 87:413–421.
12. Olin JW, Melia M, Young JR, et al. Prevalence of atherosclerotic RAS in patients with atherosclerosis elsewhere. *Am J Med* 1990; 88:46N–51N.
13. Conlon PJ, Athirakul K, Kovalik E, et al. Survival in renal vascular disease. *J Am Soc Nephrol* 1998; 9:252–256.
14. Davey Smith G, Song F, Sheldon TA. Cholesterol lowering and mortality: The importance of considering initial level of risk. *Br Med J* 1993; 306:1367–1373.
15. Adult Treatment Panel II. Summary of the second report of the National Cholesterol Education Program (NCEP) Expert Panel on the detection, evaluation and treatment of high blood cholesterol in Adults (Adult Treatment Panel II). *JAMA* 1993; 269:3015–3023.
16. Tollefson DFJ, Ernst CB. Natural history of atherosclerotic renal arterial disease associated with aortic disease. *J Vasc Surg* 1991; 14:327–331.
17. Schreiber MJ, Pohl MA, Novick AC. The natural history of atherosclerotic and fibrous renal artery disease. *Urologic Clin N Amer* 1984; 11:383–392.
18. Zierler RE, Bergelin RO, Davidson RC, et al. A prospective study of disease progression in patients with atherosclerotic renal artery stenosis. *Am J Hyper* 1996; 9:1055–1061.
19. Webster J, Marshall F, Abdalla M, et al. Randomised comparison of percutaneous angioplasty vs continued medical therapy for hypertensive patients with atheromatous renal artery stenosis. *J Hum Hypertens* 1998; 12:329–335.
20. Plouin PF, Chatellier G, Darne B, et al. Blood pressure outcome of angioplasty in atherosclerotic renal artery stenosis: A randomized trial. *Hypertension* 1998; 31:822–829.
21. Hallett JW, Textor SC, Kos PB, et al. Advanced renovascular hypertension and renal insufficiency: Trends in medical comorbidity and surgical approach from 1970 to 1993. *J Vasc Surg* 1995; 21:750–759.
22. Cambria RP, Brewster DC, L'Italien GJ, et al. Renal artery reconstruction for the preservation of renal function. *J Vasc Surg* 1996; 24:371–382.
23. Novick AC, Ziegelbaum M, Vidt DG, et al. Trends in surgical revascularization for renal artery disease: Ten years' experience. *J Urol* 1987; 257:498–501.
24. Bonelli FS, McKusick MA, Textor SC, et al. Renal artery angioplasty: Technical results and clinical outcome in 320 patients. *Mayo Clinic Proc* 1995; 70:1041–1052.
25. Tuttle KF, Chouinard RF, Webber JT, et al. Treatment of atherosclerotic ostial renal artery stenosis with the intravascular stent. *Am J Kidney Dis* 1998; 32:611–622.
26. Gross CM, Kramer J, Waigand J, et al. Ostial renal artery stent placement for atherosclerotic renal artery stenosis in patients with coronary artery disease. *Catheterization Cardiovascular Diagn* 1998; 45:1–8.
27. Chen R, Novick AC, Pohl M. Reversible renin mediated massive proteinuria successfully treated by nephrectomy. *J Urol* 1995; 153:133–134.
28. Ruggenenti P, Perna A, Benini R, et al. In chronic nephropathies prolonged ACE inhibition can induce remission: Dynamics of time-dependent changes in GFR. *J Am Soc Nephrol* 1999; 10:997–1006.
29. Ie EH, Karschner JK, Shapiro AP. Reversible nephrotic syndrome due to high renin state in renovascular hypertension. *Netherlands J Med* 1995; 46:136–141.
30. Dorros G, Jaff M, Mathiak L, et al. Four-year follow-up of Palmaz-Schatz Stent revascularization as treatment for atherosclerotic renal artery stenosis. *Circulation* 1998; 98:642–647.
31. Blum U, Krumme B, Fluegel P, et al. Treatment of ostial renal-artery stenoses with vascular endoprostheses after unsuccessful balloon angioplasty. *N Engl J Med* 1997; 336:459–465.

32. White CJ, Ramee SR, Collins TJ, et al. Renal artery stent placement: Utility in lesions difficult to treat with balloon angioplasty. *J Am Coll Cardiol* 1997; 30:1445–1450.
33. Xue F, Bettmann MA, Langdon DR, et al. Outcome and cost comparison of percutaneous transluminal renal angioplasty, renal artery stent placement, and renal arterial bypass grafting. *Radiology* 1999; 212:378–384.
34. Rundback JH, Gray RJ, Rozenblit G, et al. Renal artery stent placement for the management of ischemic nephropathy. *J Vasc Intervent Radiology* 1998; 9:413–420.
35. Harden PN, Macleod MJ, Rodger RS, et al. Effect of renal-artery stenting on progression of renovacular renal failure. *Lancet* 1997; 349:1133–1136.
36. Pohl MA, Horner C, Goormastic M, et al. Does renal revascularization preserve renal function in patients with athersclerotic renal artery stenosis? An ongoing prospective study. *J Am Soc Nephrol* 1991; 2:242–242.(Abstract)
37. Kaylor WM, Novick AC, Ziegelbaum M, et al. Reversal of end stage renal failure with surgical revascularization in patients with atherosclerotic renal artery occlusion. *J Urol* 1989; 141:486–488.
38. Hansen KJ, Starr SM, Sands RE, et al. Contemporary surgical management of renovascular disease. *J Vasc Surg* 1992; 16:319–330.
39. Lerman LO, Schwartz RS, Grande JP, et al. Noninvasive evaluation of a novel swine model of renal artery stenosis. *J Am Soc Nephrol* 1999; 10:1455–1465.
40. Steinbach F, Novick AC, Campbell S, et al. Long-term survival after surgical revascularization for atherosclerotic renal artery disease. *J Urol* 1997; 158:38–41.
41. Cambria RP, Brewster DC, L'Italien GJ, et al. The durability of different reconstructive techniques for atherosclerotic renal artery disease. *J Vasc Surg* 1994; 20:76–87.

10

Stent Revascularization of Renal Artery Stenosis:

4-Year Follow-Up of 1058 Successful Patients

Gerald Dorros, MD, Michael Jaff, DO, Lynne Mathiak, RN, and Thomas He, PhD

Introduction

Atherosclerotic renal artery stenosis may result in the new onset of or worsening blood pressure management, deterioration of renal function and loss of renal mass, recurrent pulmonary edema, or unstable angina pectoris.[1–8] In addition, renal ischemia, resulting from renal artery stenosis (RAS), has been documented to result in an absolute diminution of longitudinal kidney length.[9] These data, collected from a multicenter registry, have been collated to determine what happened to successful patients. Since patient survival appears to be adversely effected by baseline renal dysfunction despite adequate stent revascularization,[10] the cohort size in that study was relatively small (n = 145), thus, a voluntary Registry (Appendix I) was formed to clinically follow patients who had undergone successfully Palmaz stent revascularization of stenotic atherosclerotic renal arteries to further validate the previously reported observations, using the same variables of renal function, blood pressure control, and survival.[11] This chapter will detail, paraphrase, and summarize our cited publication.

From Jaff MR (ed): *Endovascular Therapy for Atherosclerotic Renal Artery Stenosis: Present and Future.* Armonk, NY: Future Publishing Co, Inc.; ©2001.

Methods

Successful Palmaz, or Palmaz-Schatz (Cordis Endovascular, Warren, NJ) stent deployment was performed in 1,058 patients in 1,443 atherosclerotic renal arteries (673 [64%] unilateral and 385 [36%] bilateral) for poorly controlled hypertension (901 patients [85%]), preservation of renal function (629 patients [59%]), and congestive heart failure (162 patients [15%]). The procedures were performed, under Institutional Review Board approved protocols, in patients with renal atherosclerotic artery stenosis, who had hypertension and/or chronic renal insufficiency, and met one or more of the following inclusion criteria: onset of hypertension after age 50 years; accelerated, severe, or malignant hypertension; inadequate response to appropriate antihypertensive therapy; poorly controlled hypertension; declining renal function after blood pressure control with pharmacologic agents; and, stenosis of one or both main renal arteries. Patients who underwent the procedure to preserve renal function had a documented serum creatinine $\geq$ 1.5 mg/dL, on two separate measurements. Procedural techniques and methodologies have been previously published.[24,33]

Follow-up data were obtained and recorded at periodic office visits such that the window for each data point at 6 months was $\pm$ 1 month, and at yearly intervals, $\pm$ 2 months. Data points outside those windows were not used. Blood pressure response was assessed by multiple observations of the systolic and diastolic pressures before and after the procedure. Renal function was assessed by serum creatinine measurements with a creatinine of >1.4 mg/dL considered abnormal and indicative of renal dysfunction. Patients were stratified into 3 groups: normal renal function ($\leq$ 1.4mg/dL; mild to moderate dysfunction (1.5 to 1.9 mg/dL); and severe dysfunction ($\geq$ 2.0 mg/dL), with a decrease in serum creatinine (> 0.2 mg/dL), representing an improvement, a value $\pm$ 0.2 mg/dL of baseline being essentially unchanged, and, an increase (> 0.2 mg/dL) being a deterioration in renal function.

Results

An atherosclerotic stenotic renal artery(s) was revascularized in 1058 patients (515 male, 543 female, mean age 69 $\pm$ 10 years) (Table 1). Procedural indications (not mutually exclusive) were poorly controlled hypertension in 901 patients (85%), preservation of renal function in 629 patients (59%) (baseline creatinine $\geq$ 1.5 mg/dL), and recurrent pulmonary edema in 62 (15%). Follow-up data (Table 2) demonstrated a durable and statistically significant improvement in blood pressure control (at 4-years: systolic: 168 $\pm$ 27 to 147 $\pm$ 21 mmHg; diastolic 84 $\pm$ 15 to 78 $\pm$ 12 mmHg; p < 0.05), as well as a significant decrease in the number of antihypertensive medications (2.4 $\pm$ 1.1 to 1.8 $\pm$ 0.9 at 3 years; p<0.05).

Creatinine levels (Tables 3 and 4), after unilateral or bilateral stent revascularization, repeatedly demonstrated a stabilization as well as significant improvement (lowering) in the serum creatinine (bilateral: 1.7 $\pm$ 1.2 to 0.8 $\pm$ 0.6;

Table 1.

Patient Demographics, Indications and Procedural Data.[b]

	Entire Cohort
Patients (Male/Female)	1058
(a) Age (yrs)	69 ±10
	Male 515 (49%)
	Female 543 (51%)
(b) Age distribution	< 70 yrs 465 (44%)
	≥ 70 yrs 593 (56%)
Procedural Indications (not mutually exclusive)	
(a) Poorly controlled hypertension	901 (85%)
(b) Preservation of renal function[a]	629 (59%)
(c) Congestive heart failure	162 (15%)
Renal Artery Stenosis	1443
(a) Unilateral Stenosis (Pts)	673 (64%)
(b) Bilateral Stenoses (Pts)	385 (36%)
Procedural Success	100%

[a]creatinine ≥ 1.5 mg/dL, [b]1,058 patients were eligible for ≥ 6 month follow-up, [c]$P < 0.05$.

Table 2.

Renal Artery Stents: 4 Year Follow-up.

Effects on Hypertension[b]	*Baseline*	*1 Yr.*	*2 Yrs.*	*3 Yrs.*	*4 Yrs.*
1. Systolic BP	168 ± 27	146 ± 24[a]	144 ± 19[a]	145 ± 22[a]	147 ± 21[a]
2. Diastolic BP	84 ± 15	75 ± 12[a]	76 ± 10[a]	76 ± 12[a]	78 ± 12[a]
3. # of Medications	2.4 ± 1.1	1.9 ± 1.0[a]	1.9 ± 1.09[a]	2.0 ± 0.9[a]	2.0 ± 1.0

[a]$P < 0.05$ paired comparison to pre value.
[b]1,058 patients were eligible for ≥ 6 month follow-up.

Table 3.

Renal Artery Stents and Effects on Renal Function: Serum Creatinine.

	Baseline	*1 Yr.*	*2 Yrs.*	*3 Yrs.*	*4 Yrs.*
Serum Creatinine (mg/dL)	1.7 ± 1.1	1.7 ± 1.2	1.3 ±1.3*	1.2 ± 0.8*	1.3 ± 0.8*

*$P < 0.05$.

Table 4.

Renal Artery Stents: Follow-up of Unilateral and Bilateral Disease Patients.

I. Changes in Serum Creatinine with Regard Unilateral and Bilateral Disease:

	Baseline	1 Yr.	2 Yrs.	3 Yrs.	4 Yrs.
a) Creatinine (mg/dL)					
i) Bilateral	1.7 ± 1.2	1.7 ± 1.1[a]	1.2 ± 1.2[a]	1.0 ± 0.8[a]	0.8 ± 0.6[a]
ii) Unilateral	1.7 ± 1.1	1.7 ± 1.2[a]	1.3 ± 1.4[a]	1.2 ± 0.8[a]	1.4 ± 0.8[a]
b) Bilateral Stenosis					
i) No change[a]	–	37%	17%	17%	8%
ii) Improved[b]	–	37%	75%	80%	92%
iii) Worse[c]	–	27%	8%	3%	0
c) Unilateral Stenosis					
i) No change[a]	–	37%	21%	22%	24%
ii) Improved[b]	–	30%	67%	67%	70%
iii) Worse[c]	–	33%	12%	9%	6%

[a]Creat. ± 0.2 mg/dL, [b]Creat. → 0.2 mg/dL, [c]Creat. → 0.2 mg/dL.

II. Effect upon Blood Pressure with Regard Unilateral or Bilateral Disease

	Baseline	1 Yr.	2 Yrs.	3 Yrs.	4 Yrs.
1. Bilateral Stenosis					
Systolic BP (mmHg)	167 ± 28	144 ± 24*	143 ± 18*	142 ± 17*	140 ± 19*
Diastolic BP (mmHg)	83 ± 15	74 ± 12[a]	74 ± 10[a]	74 ± 9[a]	75 ± 12[a]
# Meds	2.5 ± 1.1	2.0 ± 1.1*	1.9 ± 1.0*	1.7 ± 0.9	1.9 ± 1.1
2. Unilateral Stenosis					
Systolic BP (mmHg)	168 ± 27	147 ± 25*	145 ± 20*	146 ± 23*	149 ± 22*
Diastolic BP (mmHg)	85 ± 15	76 ± 12	77 ± 10[a]	77 ± 12[a]	79 ± 12
# Meds	2.4 ± 1.1	1.8 ± 1.0[a]	1.9 ± 1.2	1.9 ± 0.9	2.0 ± 1.0

[a]$p < 0.05$.

and unilateral: 1.7 ± 1.1 to 1.4 ± 0.8; $p < 0.05$). Furthermore, 70% of unilateral and 92% of bilateral patients had stabilization or improved function, and relatively few patients had a worsening of renal function.

The 4-year cumulative probability of survival for all patients was 74% ± 3%, with few deaths related to end-stage renal disease. Patients with unilateral disease had a 75% ± 3% survival, which was not statistically different than the 70% ± 5% survival of patients with bilateral disease (Table 5). Survival was adversely influenced ($p < 0.05$) by both worsening renal function, and was especially adversely influenced by bilateral renal artery stenosis and severe renal dysfunction (creatinine ≥ 2.0 mg/dl), despite successful stent revascularization. Patients with mild to moderate renal dysfunction had a survival probability of 78% ± 7% if the stenosis were unilateral, and 78% ± 7% ($p < 0.05$) if bilateral. Patients with severe baseline renal dysfunction had a 49% ± 5% survival; furthermore, the presence of bilateral disease significantly adversely impacted survival (unilateral: 55% ± 6% vs. bilateral: 36% ± 11%; $p < 0.05$).

Table 5.

Renal Stent Follow-up: Survival as Related to Baseline Creatinine, and Extent of Renal Artery Stenosis.

		Survival Probability at 4 Yrs.	
	Entire Cohort	*Unilateral Disease*	*Bilateral Disease*
1. Baseline Creatinine (mg/dL)			
≤1.4	85% ± 3% (622)	86% ± 3% (397)	85% ± 7% (225)
1.5 – 1.9	78% ± 5%[a] (168)	78% ± 7% (103)	78% ± 7% (65)
≥ 2.0	49% ± 5%[a] (268)	55% ± 6% (173)	36% ± 11% (95)
2. Anatomy	74% ± 3% (1,058)	75% ± 3% (673)	70% ± 5% (385)
3. Age			
≥ 70 years	66% ± 24% (593)	–	–
< 70 years	82% ± 3% (465)[a]	–	–
4. Procedural Indication			
Poorly controlled BP	77% ± 3% (901)	–	–
Controlled BP	57% ± 8% (148)[a]	–	–

[a]$P < 0.05.$

Discussion

Atherosclerotic renal artery stenosis occurs frequently in patients with mild or moderate hypertension, end-stage renal disease, and diffuse atherosclerosis; and, this obstructive process is progressive: stenoses become occlusions[3,4] in approximately 15% of cases, renal function deteriorates in 10%–20% of cases,[4] and the more severe the initial stenosis, the more likely progression to occlusion.[3] Untreated renal artery stenosis has been correlated with a loss of renal mass.[9] Furthermore, the first manifestation of renal artery stenosis can be an evident cardiac dysfunction: flash pulmonary edema, congestive heart failure, or unstable angina.[7,8]

Renal artery stent revascularization procedural results have been demonstrated to be superior to balloon angioplasty,[12] as assessed by hemodynamic transstenotic pressure gradient measurements, complication rates, and restenosis rates. The data herein define its long-term benefits as manifest by significant decreases in the systolic and diastolic blood pressures, more facile blood pressure control, a reduction in the number of antihypertensive medications, and overall improvement in renal function. Actuarial analysis demonstrated that impaired baseline renal function and/or bilateral disease adversely influenced survival. However, these data more clearly detail what happens to patients after stent revascularization, and while often in concert with Dorros' publications,[10,13] do provide further elucidation. This large cohort's data demonstrate a much more beneficial effect upon renal function both with regard to stabilization or improvement in serum creatinine levels. Thus, fewer patients had a worsening of renal function, as was previously reported,[10] which modifies, somewhat, the concern that this procedure could adversely impact patients who had normal renal function and severely stenotic atherosclerotic renal arteries. Furthermore, the beneficial effect upon blood pressure, coupled with a diminution in the number of antihypertensive drugs could significantly impact survival. Finally, the recent publication[9] detailing the correlation between RAS and kidney atrophy, coupled with the small risk of worsening renal function by stent revascularization,[10] makes this procedure even more appealing.

Conclusions

Revascularization of stenotic atherosclerotic renal arteries was effectively achieved with balloon expandable Palmaz-Schatz™ stents in 1,058 patients, and their follow-up clinical data substantiated published conclusions concerning stent revascularization's effect upon renal function, blood pressure control, and survival. Furthermore, this large patient cohort provided clarification about the follow-up results in patient subsets. However, the cumulative probability of survival of patients with severe renal insufficiency was dismal when compared to those patients with normal, mild, or moderate impairment in baseline renal function, and the patient outcome worsened with bilaterality of disease.

While the appropriate treatment of RAS may be as yet not agreed upon, the failure to diagnosis RAS before end-organ damage has occurred really appears not to be a moot point. Since RAS appears to be a readily amenable condition, simply and safely managed with stent-supported angioplasty, the failure of a physician to not consider its diagnosis seems unacceptable.

Stent revascularization appears not only preferential to surgical alternatives in patients with an anticipated increased surgical risk, on the sole basis of surgical morbidity and mortality rates, but could be, as well, for patients with asymptomatic (normal blood pressure and serum creatinine levels) renal artery stenosis. However, the latter concept requires a more focused study. Stent revascularization, with its gratifying success rates, acceptable procedural risks, beneficial impact upon blood pressure control and renal function, as well as the excellent follow-up results in patients with normal baseline renal function, make it the procedure of choice for atherosclerotic renal artery stenosis.

APPENDIX I.

List of participants in Multicenter Registry

1. Dorros G, Mathiak LM, He T. Dorros-Feuer Interventional Cardiovascular Disease Foundation, Grafton, WI and Phoenix, AZ
2. Jaff M. The Heart and Vascular Institute, Morristown, NJ
3. Ramee S, McCarthy R. Ochsner Medical Institution, New Orleans, LA

4. Diethrich EB, Rodrigues J. Arizona Heart Institute, Phoenix, AZ
5. Minor R, Harner R, Pensabene R, Nautiyal, Wedgebury L, Berstein R, Straw S, Krause E. Rockford Cardiology Associates, Rockford, IL
6. Krajcer Z. Texas Heart Institute, Houston, TX
7. Rosenfield K. St. Elizabeth's Medical Center, Boston, MA
8. Piegari R, Atkinson, L. Berks Cardiologists, Reading, PA

References

1. Wollenweber J, Sheps SG, Davis GD. Clinical course of atherosclerotic vascular disease. *Am J Cardiol* 1968; 21:60–71.
2. Meaney TF, Dustan HP, McCormack LJ. Natural history of renal artery disease. *Radiology* 1968; 91:881–887.
3. Schreiber MJ, Pohl MA, Novick AC. The natural history of atherosclerotic and fibrous renal artery disease. *Urol Clin North Am* 1984; 11:383–392.
4. Rimmer JM, Gennari FJ. Atherosclerotic renovascular disease and progressive renal failure. *Ann Intern Med* 1993; 118:712–719.
5. Mailloux LU. Atherosclerotic renovascular disease causing end-stage renal disease: The case for earlier diagnosis and therapy. *J Vasc Med Biol* 1993; 4:277–284.
6. Mailloux LU, Napolitano B, Bellucci AG, et al. Renal vascular disease causing end-stage renal disease, incidence, clinical correlates, and outcomes: A 20-year clinical experience. *Am J Kidney Diseases* 1994; 24:622–629.
7. Pickering TG, Herman L, Devereux RB, et al. Recurrent pulmonary edema in hypertension due to bilateral renal artery stenosis: Treatment by angioplasty of surgical revascularization. *Lancet* 1988; 2:551–552.
8. Messena LM, Zelenock GB, Yao KA, Stanley SC. Renal revascularization for recurrent pulmonary edema in patients with poorly controlled hypertension and renal insufficiency. A distinct subgroup of patients with atherosclerotic renal artery occlusive disease. *J Vasc Surg* 1992; 15:73–82.
9. Caps MT, Zierler RE, Polissar N, et al. Risk of atrophy in kidneys with atherosclerotic renal artery stenosis. *Kidney International* 1998; 53:735–742.
10. Dorros G, Jaff M, Mathiak L, et al. Four-year follow-up of Palmaz-Schatz stent revascularization as treatment for atherosclerotic renal artery stenosis. *Circulation* 1998; 98: 642–647.
11. Dorros G, Jaff M, Mathiak L, et al. Multicenter Palmaz™ Stent Renal Artery Stenosis Revascularization Registry: 4-year follow-up of 1058 successful patients. *Cathet Cardiovasc Diagn* (submitted for publication)
12. Dorros G, Jaff M, Jain A, et al. Follow-up of primary Palmaz-Schatz stent placement for atherosclerotic renal artery stenosis. *Am J Cardiol* 1995; 75:1051–1055.
13. Dorros G, Prince CR, Mathiak LM. Stenting of a renal artery stenosis achieves better relief of the obstructive lesion than balloon angioplasty. *Cathet Cardiovasc Diagn* 1993; 29:191–198.

Subject Index

Page numbers followed by "t" indicate tables.